GROOMING MANUAL FOR THE DOG AND CAT

Sue Dallas VN, Cert Ed
Diana North GCGI
Joanne Angus LCGI

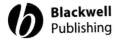

Blackwell
Publishing

Editorial offices:
Blackwell Publishing Ltd, 9600 Garsington Road, Oxford OX4 2DQ, UK
  Tel: +44 (0) 1865 776868
Blackwell Publishing Professional, 2121 State Avenue, Ames, Iowa 50014-8300, USA
  Tel: +1 515 29 20140
Blackwell Publishing Asia Pty Ltd, 550 Swanston Street, Carlton, Victoria 3053, Australia
  Tel: +61 (0)3 8359 1011

First published 2006 by Blackwell Publishing Ltd

ISBN 978-1-4051-1183-6

Library of Congress Cataloging-in-Publication Data
Dallas, S.E. (Sue E.)
   Grooming manual for the dog and cat/Sue Dallas, Diana North, Joanne Angus.
       p.   cm.
   Includes bibliographical references and index.
   ISBN 978-1-4051-1183-6 (pbk. : alk. paper)
     1. Dogs–Grooming.   2. Cats–Grooming.   I. North, Diana.   II. Angus, Joanne.
III. Title. \

SF427.5D35 2006
636.7'08'33–dc22
2005022934

A catalogue record for this title is available from the British Library

Set in 10/12.5 pt Palatino
by Graphicraft Limited, Hong Kong

The publisher's policy is to use permanent paper from mills that operate a sustainable forestry policy, and which has been manufactured from pulp processed using acid-free and elementary chlorine-free practices. Furthermore, the publisher ensures that the text paper and cover board used have met acceptable environmental accreditation standards.

For further information on Blackwell Publishing, visit our website:
www.blackwellpublishing.com

Printed in the UK

Contents

Preface

The pet-owning population is growing, and with it the need for technical and practical knowledge of grooming and care of pets.

It is against the background of increasing growth in pet ownership and showing that the authors decided to write this book. It contains information on the breeds and coat types of dogs and cats, pre-grooming and general care and detailed step-by-step grooming and clipping techniques. The allied chapters to grooming contain useful information on skin and skin conditions, canine and feline diseases, parasites and first aid.

The dogs and cats featured in this book are a mix of pet and show animals to give the reader the opportunity to see the differences in grooming styles.

Both the professional groomer and the pet owner have been catered for in the easy-to-use format. The authors hope this book is useful to those starting a career in grooming, working towards a qualification in animal and nursing care, and as a reference text for grooming salons.

Many thanks go to the staff at Blackwell Publishing for their support throughout this project. Thanks also go to our colleagues, friends and families for giving us their support and encouragement to complete this book, particularly Peter, David and Leon.

Sue Dallas
Diana North
Joanne Angus

Acknowledgements

Our thanks are due to:

David Crossley, who took the photographs of the salon dogs and equipment.

Carolyn Lowing, of Pet Mentors, who created the sketches and contributed to the sections on dog behaviour.

Carol Flatt of Dezynadog, for contributing to the chapter on equipment care and for allowing us the run of their new premises and equipment.

Alison Thomas and David North for all their support and encouragement.

Competitors at Eurogroom 2005.

The customers and dogs at Look North Grooming and Training Centre Ltd.

The authors thank the following for their permission to reproduce materials used in this book:

The Kennel Club for extracts from the Breeds Standards.

John D. Jackson, photographer, for a selection of his breed photographs.

Mary Allen for photographs in Chapter 1.

About the Authors

Sue Dallas is a qualified veterinary nurse, and has worked in veterinary schools and veterinary practices in the UK and in North America. She has taught on both veterinary nursing and animal care courses for over 20 years and has been involved in a number of educational and examination developments. Sue has spoken at veterinary congresses both in the UK and around the world, promoting nursing and care of animals through training and education. In the early 1990s she became Editor of the *Veterinary Nursing Journal*, the official journal of the British Veterinary Nursing Association, and has also published textbooks for animal carers, veterinary nurses and auxiliary nurses.

Diana North and Joanne Angus have worked together in grooming for over 25 years and won many competitions both in the UK and abroad. As a salon, they specialised in training for groomers starting in the industry, pet owners and those wishing to improve their skills. Their company was the first grooming business to achieve the Investors in People award in 1995 and has continued to meet the national standards through the re-recognition process.

Joanne owns the Look North Grooming and Training Centre Ltd. She is an Advanced Groomer and a founder member of the Guild of Advanced Groomers. She has been Groomer of the Year on two occasions and won Best in Show at Eurogroom and a Gold Medal at Intergroom, USA. She is an examiner for the 7750 NPTC City and Guilds Advanced Certificate in Dog Grooming and the Pet Care Trust's BDGA Higher Diploma in Dog Grooming.

Diana is now retired from hands-on grooming but continues to be part of the education side of the industry. She is an External Verifier for the National Vocational Qualifications in Animal Care and a regular speaker to groomers groups about the 7750 NPTC City and Guilds Advanced Certificate. She also spends time generally giving guidance on career routes in grooming. Diana is a founder member of the Guild of Advanced Groomers and an examiner for the grooming qualifications, having worked over the years on their development. Diana also answers grooming questions for *Your Dog* magazine.

Part 1
What You Need To Know

Breed Groups and Coat Types

DOGS

In this book we will be describing the specific pet and breed grooming styles for the commonest breeds seen today.

There are many different ways to categorise the dog breeds seen in the UK: by size, colour, characteristics or coat type. We shall be using two systems in this book, which have been cross-referenced to help you find your way through the many breeds.

- System one – Kennel Club breed groupings
- System two – Coat types

The breed groups

The Kennel Club categorises breeds into seven groups: Gundogs, Hounds, Pastoral, Terriers, Toy, Utility and Working. It helps while grooming a dog to bear in mind what it was originally bred for.

The Gundog group

Gundogs are quite natural looking, bred to work in the field or water. They are used to hunt, point and retrieve. In this group we find many of the commonest breeds seen today — Golden Retrievers, Labradors, Setters and Spaniels (Fig. 1.1).

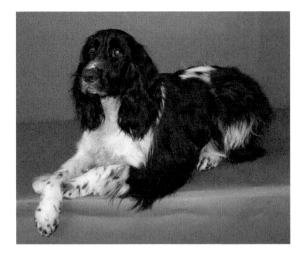

Fig. 1.1 Springer Spaniel.

The Hound group

Hounds use either sight or scent for hunting purposes and therefore may be very independent. They vary hugely in their construction from the small, low to ground Miniature Dachshund to the giant Irish Wolfhound. Fig. 1.2 shows an Afghan Hound.

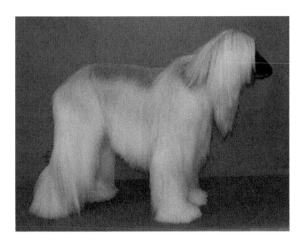

Fig. 1.2 Afghan Hound.

The Pastoral group

These are the shepherding and herding breeds that are used worldwide to keep flocks and herds under control. The Border Collie, German Shepherd (Fig. 1.3) and Old English Sheepdog are some examples.

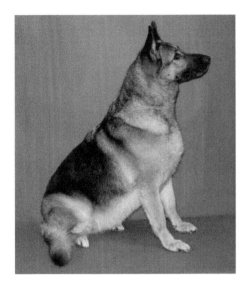

Fig. 1.3 German Shepherd.

The Terrier group

Terriers are the ratters and vermin hunters, very keen and sometimes wilful. They are often easily categorised by their distinct harsh coats (Fig. 1.4) but there are some in the group who differ, such as the Bedlington and Kerry Blue.

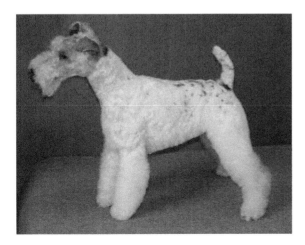

Fig. 1.4 Wire Fox Terrier.

The Toy group

These are the companion dogs sought after for their 'knee-warming' skills but don't be misled into believing that they do not have the same character as some of their bigger relations. This group contains breeds such as the Yorkshire Terrier, Bichon Frise (Fig. 1.5) and Cavalier King Charles Spaniel.

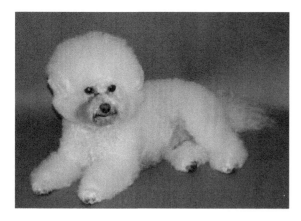

Fig. 1.5 Bichon Frise.

The Utility group

This is a vastly mixed group of dogs each with their own character or working abilities. They range from the Poodle to the Miniature Schnauzer to the Lhasa Apso (Fig. 1.6).

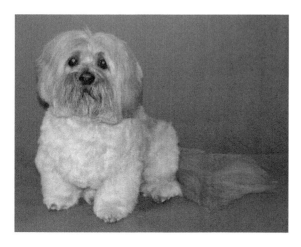

Fig. 1.6 Lhasa Apso.

The Working group

The breeds in this group include the guarders and defenders. The commonest ones are the Dobermann (Fig. 1.7) and Rottweiler and then come the giant breeds such as St. Bernard and Newfoundland.

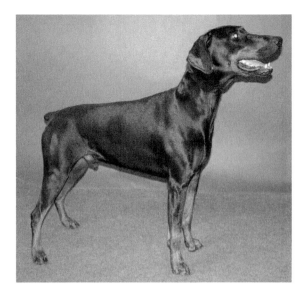

Fig. 1.7 Dobermann.

Coat types

For ease of reference we have categorised coats into five types: double coat, silky coat, smooth coat, wire coat and wool coat.

Double coats

A double coat consists of a dense, soft undercoat concealed by a longer topcoat. Several breeds of dog fit this coat type, so for the purposes of this book we have split this group into two:

- Double coat — one (untrimmed or tidied). The breeds with this type of coat are those that require much grooming and removal of dead undercoat with little or no trimming. Examples are the German Shepherd, Rough Collie, Samoyed, St. Bernard and Tervueren (Fig. 1.8).
- Double coat — two (trimmed). These breeds have a much longer topcoat, which in theory (and particularly for show purposes) should not be trimmed. However, for pet purposes a more practical, shortened style is far more appropriate. Examples are the Lhasa Apso (Fig. 1.9), Shih Tzu and Old English Sheepdog.

Silky coat

The most important feature of this coat is its texture and not the length. Once again, breeds with this type of coat may require a lot or a small amount of trimming. Breed examples include the Afghan Hound, spaniels such as the Cavalier King Charles Spaniel (Fig. 1.10) and Yorkshire Terrier.

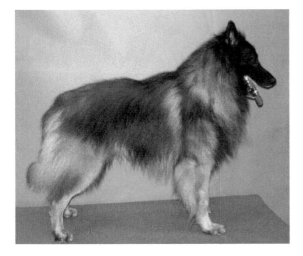

Fig. 1.8 Tervueren.

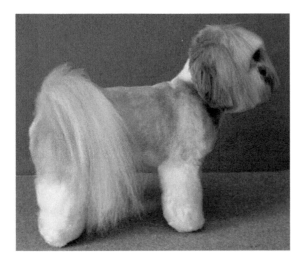

Fig. 1.9 Lhasa Apso in teddy bear trim.

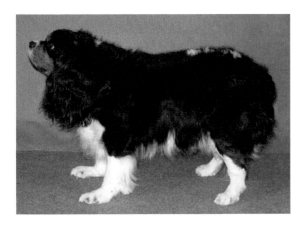

Fig. 1.10 King Charles Spaniel.

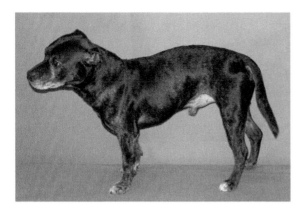

Fig. 1.11 Staffordshire Bull Terrier.

Smooth coat

This coat is easily defined by the length, being short and tight to the body. This coat type is the low-maintenance type in grooming terms. The main objectives of grooming these breeds is to remove dead coat and give a glossy finish. Breed examples include the Boxer, Dobermann, Weimeraner and the Staffordshire Bull Terrier (Fig. 1.11).

Wire coat

This coat has a harsh, dense topcoat with a softer undercoat. The coat should be 'hand-stripped' to maintain the correct texture and colour but many pets are clipped for the ease and cost of grooming – this is not acceptable in the show ring. The main breed examples here are terriers, e.g. West Highland White, Wire Fox, Border (Fig. 1.12) and Scottish Terrier although there are other breeds such as the Miniature Schnauzer and Wire Haired Dachshund.

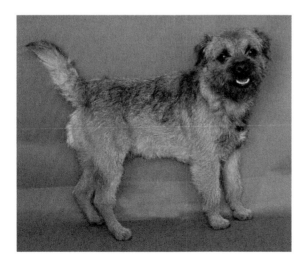

Fig. 1.12 Border Terrier.

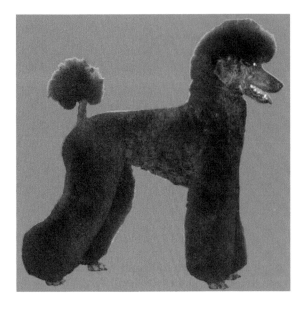

Fig. 1.13 Standard Poodle.

Wool coat

For the purpose of this book we have used this group to include a multitude of breeds whose coats perhaps fit better here than under other coat types, although Breed Standards do not specify 'wool coat'. These breeds require specific drying techniques and trimming styles. Examples are poodles (Fig. 1.13), Irish Water Spaniels and Bichon (Fig. 1.5).

Irrespective of breed or coat type, all dogs should be groomed on a regular basis for many reasons:

- Promotes good handler—dog relationship.
- Promotes health, cleanliness and well-being of the dog.
- Provides an opportunity to inspect the dog for any skin, coat or health problems.

Always remember that when you are grooming a dog you are the one in charge and not the dog. Learn to make grooming a pleasurable experience for both you and the dog. Further details of handling are covered in Chapter 4.

Cross-reference system

The breeds are in alphabetical order with their breed group represented as follows:

Gd = Gundogs   To = Toy
Ho = Hounds   Ut = Utility
Pa = Pastoral   Wo = Working
Te = Terriers

The coat types will also be abbreviated as follows:

Dc1 = Double coat — one	Dc2 = Double coat — two
Si = Silky	Sm = Smooth
Wi = Wire	Wo = Wool

Gundogs *(Gd)*

English Setter	Si
Gordon Setter	Si
Irish Setter	Si
Italian Spinone	Wi
Retriever	
Flat Coat	Dc1
Golden	Dc1
Labrador	Dc1
Spaniels	
American Cocker	Si
Clumber	Si
Cocker	Si
English Springer	Si
Field	Si
Irish Water	Wo
Sussex	Si
Welsh Springer	Si

Hounds *(Ho)*

Afghan	Si
Dachshund	Sm, Wi or Si
Deerhound	Wi
Irish Wolfhound	Wi

Pastoral *(Pa)*

Bearded Collie	Dc2
Border Collie	Dc1 or Sm
German Shepherd	Dc1
Old English Sheepdog	Dc2
Polish Lowland Sheepdog	Dc2
Rough Collie	Dc1
Samoyed	Dc1
Shetland Sheepdog	Dc1

Terriers *(Te)*

Airedale	Wi
Bedlington	Wo
Border	Wi
Cairn	Wi
Dandie Dinmont	Wi
Irish	Wi
Kerry Blue	Si
Lakeland	Wi
Norfolk	Wi
Norwich	Wi
Parson Russell Terrier	Wi
Scottish	Wi
Sealyham	Wi
Soft Coated Wheaten	Si
Welsh	Wi
West Highland White	Wi
Wire Fox	Wi

Toys *(To)*

Bichon Frise	Wo
Cavalier King Charles Spaniel	Si
Griffon Bruxellois	Wi or Sm
Lowchen	Si
Maltese	Si
Papillion	Si
Pekingese	Dc1
Pomeranian	Dc1
Yorkshire Terrier	Si

Utility *(Ut)*

Chow Chow	Dc1
Lhasa Apso	Dc2
Miniature Schnauzer	Wi
Poodle	Wo
Schnauzer	Wi
Shih Tzu	Dc2
Tibetan Terrier	Dc2

Working *(Wo)*

Bernese Mountain Dog	Dc1
Bouvier des Flandres	Dc2

Boxer	Sm
Dobermann	Sm
Giant Schnauzer	Wi
Newfoundland	Dc1
St. Bernard	Dc1

Of course there are some exceptionally different coats in the world of dogs, which we felt needed a mention, such as the corded coat of the Hungarian Puli and the unusual look of the Chinese Crested. However, specialist knowledge is required for maintaining the coats of these breeds and therefore these are not covered in this book.

In Chapter 2 the breed names are followed by the group and coat type's abbreviated name so that you know which tools and equipment are relevant for each, for example:

- Bernese Mountain Dog (Wo-Dc1) = Working dog with Double coat — one.
- West Highland White (Te-Wi) = Terrier group with a wire coat.

Working with this book should be easy, as specific details for trimming each breed are given on a designated page (see Chapter 11). There are sections on grooming out, and bathing and drying in Chapters 4, 6 and 9, and these are reinforced in the checklists in Chapter 10 and the breed profiles in Chapter 11. In cases of breeds with similar trimming requirements, cross-references have been provided to the other breed(s).

CATS

A cat's fur is its most admired feature, and it is also an important part of its body. It is not just the basis for cat breed identification but on a functional level it:

- Provides a barrier between the cat's skin and its environment
- Protects the cat from injury and infection
- Helps to regulate body temperature
- Insulates the body in cold weather
- Is a general guide to health
- Protects against excess sunlight and chemicals

The coat hair may be:

- Long
- Short
- Hard
- Soft
- Silky
- Coarse
- Thick
- Wavy

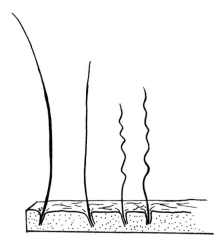

Fig. 1.14 Cat hair types. From left to right: guard, awn and down hair.

Selective breeding and genetic mutation have enhanced cats' coats and in fact have caused coat loss. The result is that the various cat breeds not only have different textures of coat but also have an incredible variety of colour and coat pattern. The basic type of cat, the wild type, is the Tabby cat. It is from the Tabby that all other breeds of cat have evolved. A cat's coat may contain up to 200 hairs per square millimetre (130 000 per square inch). The cat has a top coat of guard hair and an undercoat which consists of coarse, bristly awn hairs and soft down hairs (Fig. 1.14).

The guard or primary hairs normally form the coarse outer layer of the coat. In the cat these hairs tend to be rooted in individual hair follicles. They are connected to the nervous system (autonomic) and therefore respond to information from the senses (eyes, ears, smell and touch) in the form of excitement, fear, cold or the fight reflex. The guard hairs stand upright at these times giving the cat an aggressive appearance. There are more of these hairs on the cat's back and sides making it appear larger to another animal. If the cat is cold then these hairs stand up providing an area around the cat in which to trap body heat and thus acts as a form of insulation. Throughout the top coat of guard hairs is the under coat made up of bristly awn hairs with thickened tips and the soft downy hairs which lie close to the skin.

Generally cats are considered to be either short haired or long haired with a guard hair length from 4.5 cm to 15 cm. Besides the length, there is the coat's density and texture. This is provided by the guard, awn, and down hairs. These three hairs vary from one breed to another.

The ideal coat of a pedigree cat has been set out in Breed and Show Standards, over the last 100 years of selective breeding. The aim of the Standards is to ensure that any proposed new breed is different from other registered breeds and that there are enough potential breeders interested in breeding the cat to support the agreed Standard. The process may take a number of years, through preliminary and provisional stages before being shown in championship level classes. This is regulated by the Governing Council of the Cat Fancy.

For grooming purposes, cat breeds can be subdivided into:

- Long hair: Persian
- Semi-long hair: Birman, Turkish Van, Ragdoll
- Short hair: British short hair, Manx
- Short hair: Foreign Abyssinian, Russian Blue, Cornish and Devon Rex
- Short hair: American Shaded Silver, Red Tabby
- Burmese: Burmese
- Oriental: Oriental Black, Blue and Caramel Havana
- Siamese: Siamese, Balinese

In North America domestic cats are categorised in two groups only:

- Long hair
- Short hair

Coat types

Long coat

Cats with long coats have large bodies and a round head. The nose is short, the eyes are large and the ears are small. The coat is long and double with soft undercoat and quite coarse guard hairs of almost the same length as the undercoat (Fig. 1.15). Although these cats will self-groom, to prevent matting of the coat the owner needs to assist the cat. This will prevent tangles forming, which the cat cannot deal with. Typical long haired breeds include Persian and Angora.

In the long hair coat the down hair is almost as long as the guard hair, giving the coat a soft silky feel. The longest guard hair length is about 12.5 cm (Fig. 1.16). Breeds like the Turkish or Birman, though genetically the same as the Persian, have shorter down hairs, leaving the coat less full.

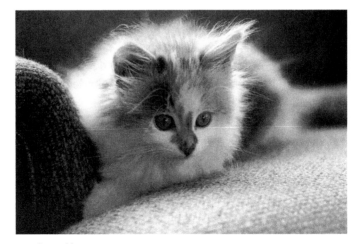

Fig. 1.15 Long-haired kitten.

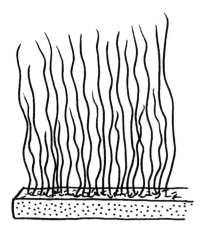

Fig. 1.16 Long hair and semi-long hair with guard hairs which may exceed 12.5 cm and down hairs of various lengths.

Semi-long coat

These cats are sturdy and muscular with a normal shaped head and length of nose. The eyes are of normal size, however the upright ears can be large. The coat is long but not as double as the Persian, having either a finer or a shaggy texture (which means that the coat is less liable to matting).

Short coat

This coat is dense and easy to care for. It is easier to clean and unlikely to get tangled. Fig. 1.17 a and b show cats with typical short coats. Fig. 1.18 is a diagrammatic illustration of how short hair grows.

  These cats' features vary depending on their origin, for example:

- British Shorthair: These cats have a stocky build, with large round heads and muscular body and short legs.
- American Shorthair: These cats are larger than the British/European breeds, with a lean body. They are longer legged with an oval head.
- Foreign Shorthair: These cats are slim bodied and long legged, their coat contains fine hairs and the head is wedge shaped.

Curly or wavy coat

The curly or wavy coat has either no guard hair or very short guard hair (see also Chapter 5). It comprises short curly awn and down hairs that are of the same length, giving the coat a curly, wavy appearance, e.g. the Cornish Rex (Fig. 1.19). The Devon Rex coat has all three types of hair, however the guard and awn are so altered they resemble down hairs giving the coat a harsher feel. The Devon Rex also varies in that it has either shortened whiskers or none at all.

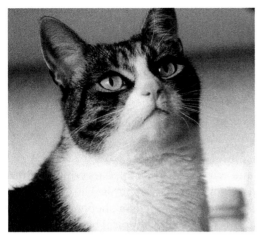

(a)

Fig. 1.17 (a) Short-haired cat (I).
(b) Short-haired cat (II).

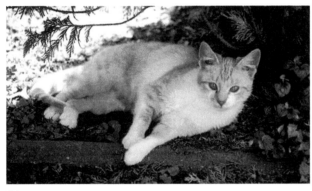

(b)

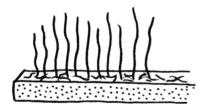

Fig. 1.18 Short hair is the normal or wild type, with the longest guard hair of about 4.5 cm.

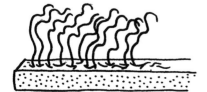

Fig. 1.19 The curly coat has no guard hairs with natural curls in the awn and down hairs.

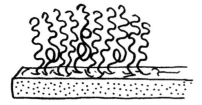

Fig. 1.20 Wire coat contains all types of hair abnormally curled, the awn hair looking like a shepherd's crook.

Wire coat

The coat is thick, curly, woolly, coarse and wiry to touch. It appears crimped due to the wave or curl of the hairs, and some are even coiled in spirals. The guard hair and down are similar, the tips of the awn hair looking like a shepherd's crook, with some even coiled into complete spirals (Fig. 1.20). A typical breed with this coat type is the American Blue Wirehair.

Hairless

These cats do in fact have some hairs, but they are so sparse that the appearance is hairless. Down hairs around the face, legs and body give a thin covering (1.21). With little or no hair to protect the skin and help in body heat conservation this breed needs assistance in cold weather and early treatment for any obvious skin damage. The skin and down hair can be of any recognised colour and pattern, such as that seen in the Blue Sphynx (1.22).

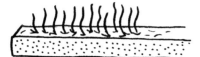

Fig. 1.21 The hairless coat has a thin covering of down hair.

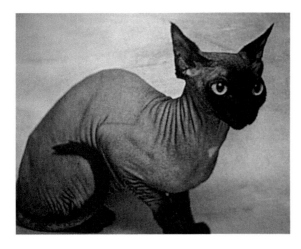

Fig. 1.22 The Sphynx cat.

Equipment and Techniques

There are many different makes and types of grooming equipment available to enable you to do your work well. 'A bad workman always blames his tools' is an old quotation; however, we believe 'You need the right tools to do a good job'. Don't be tempted to think that 'cheapest is best' even if you are just buying a brush and comb for your pet. If you buy good-quality products they will, with correct use, last you a long time and produce the results required.

BRUSHES

In general for all coat types except smooth coats, a slicker brush (Fig. 2.1) is the most useful tool. Always be aware when purchasing a new slicker that the pins will be quite hard and will need to be 'worn in'. Over-use of the slicker brush can cause abrasion of the skin known as 'slicker burn' or 'brush burn'. This can potentially lead to more severe skin problems as the dog will lick and chew the affected

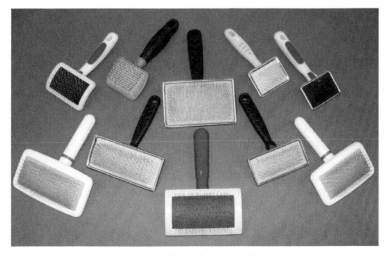

Fig. 2.1 Selection of slicker brushes: note the wide variety of sizes and colours.

area, and secondary infection could follow. Therefore correct usage of the brush is important.

Hold the brush lightly and place the fingers as shown in Fig. 2.2. Holding the brush in this way decreases the chance of slicker burn. Always brush from the bottom layers of the coat outwards to ensure that you are getting down to the bottom of the coat (Fig. 2.3) and not just brushing over the topcoat and neglecting the undercoat. This is particularly important for coat types Dc1, Dc2 and Wo.

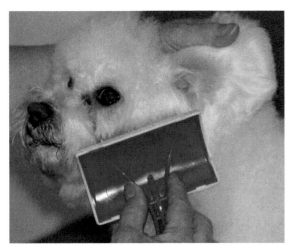 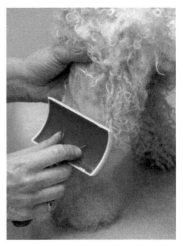

Fig. 2.2 (*Left*) Hold the slicker brush lightly and place the fingers as shown.
Fig. 2.3 (*Right*) When using the slicker brush, hold the coat in sections to get to the base (undercoat).

In breeds such as the Lhasa Apso (Ut-Dc2) and Old English Sheepdog (Pa-Dc2), which should have a long coat for show purposes, a slicker brush is not appropriate because the brush will break and tear the coat. For the correct maintenance of the coat texture of these coat types, a pin or bristle brush should be used (Fig. 2.4). These brushes are much softer than the slicker, but a great deal of practice is required to use them correctly otherwise the coat will not be groomed to the skin.

For smooth-coated breeds, a rubber brush or glove is an excellent tool for removing the dead undercoat and creating a shiny top/outer coat (Fig. 2.5).

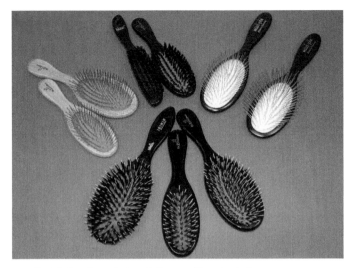

Fig. 2.4 Pin and bristle brushes: choice of sizes and length of pins.

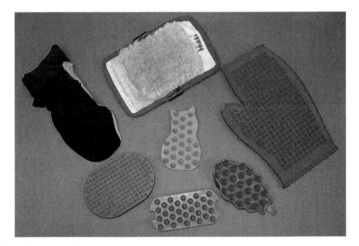

Fig. 2.5 Hand gloves, rubber brushes and terrier pad.

COMBS

A good general-purpose comb is one of medium length with medium width teeth at one end and finer teeth at the other. This comb will suit all coat types except for smooth coats. Smooth coats require very little combing although a flea comb is useful for getting out those ultra-fine dead hairs. For longer coats, e.g. in Bearded Collies (Pa-Dc2) or Afghan Hounds (Ho-Si), you may find that a wider, longer tooth comb is more useful to get down to the bottom of the coat (Figs 2.6 and 2.7).

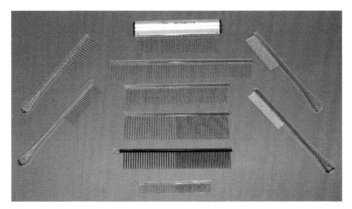

Fig. 2.6 Selection of combs with or without handles: note the wide variety of the length of the teeth.

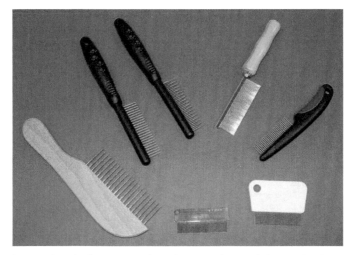

Fig. 2.7 Selection of combs from very wide teeth to very close and short teeth. There is also a flea comb.

Always ensure that you have thoroughly brushed the coat before using the comb, as the comb will pull the tangles and cause discomfort to the dog (Figs 2.8 and 2.9).

Imagine grooming your own hair – brush first to remove tangles and then comb through to ensure completely knot-free hair.

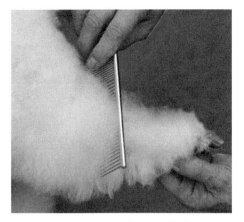

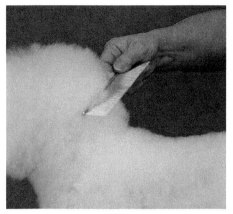

Fig. 2.8 Using the comb to check after brushing.

Fig. 2.9 Using the comb to lift and separate a wool coat.

DE-MATTING TOOLS

Various de-matting tools are available on the market (Fig. 2.10) but the one favoured by many professional groomers is the 'Mikki Mat Breaker'. When using de-matting tools remember that the teeth are blades and can cut skin. Always use the de-matter to break through knots, not to rip them out. In severely matted coats you can try to brush open the mats first and then ease the de-matter through, and then brush again to remove the knots. Take care around the ears, especially in breeds such as the Cocker Spaniel (Gu-Si), as it is very easy to tear the skin in this area. If the mats are very close and tight to the skin then no de-matting tool will remove them. It will be much safer for the dog if you use a clipper (Fig. 2.11) to remove these mats, thus eliminating the chances of injury.

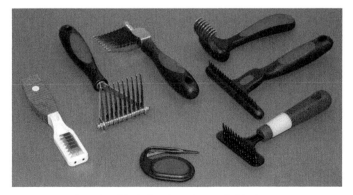

Fig. 2.10 De-matting tools: rakes, bladed tools and a single blade.

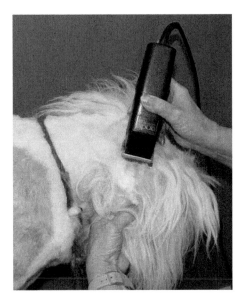

Fig. 2.11 Use the clipper to remove mats around the ear.

COAT KINGS

Coat Kings are a relatively new product on the market (Fig. 2.12). These tools are proving to be an invaluable addition to the professional dog owner/groomer's toolbox. They come with a range of replaceable blade sizes from 6 to 33 blades. There is a selection of mini and jumbo blades. The wider teeth can be used for thinning out coats of breeds from the Dc1 group, the medium sizes are most useful for silky coats which have become fluffy, and the narrow teeth tools are most useful for wire coats, aiding hand-stripping. However, take care not to over use this tool or you may remove too much coat.

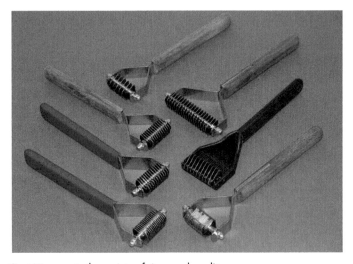

Fig. 2.12 Coat Kings: note the variety of sizes and quality.

STRIPPING EQUIPMENT

Hand-stripping is a technique which should be used on wire coats and some silky coats to maintain the correct coat texture and colour. Examples of breeds this applies to are Airedale Terrier (Te-Wi), Giant Schnauzer (Wo-Wi) and Irish Setter (Gd-Si).

Using the finger and thumb is the best stripping method (Fig. 2.13): it is readily available and ensures that there is no cutting of the coat.

There is a huge variety of stripping knives (Fig. 2.14), although the term 'knife' is something of a misnomer as they should not cut the coat but just act as an aid to hand-stripping.

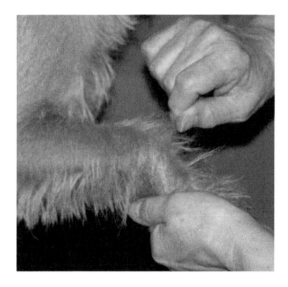

Fig. 2.13 Using the finger and thumb to hand-strip the coat.

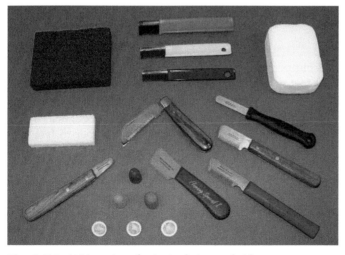

Fig. 2.14 Wide variety of stripping knives and aids.

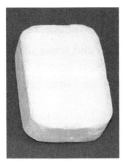

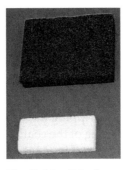

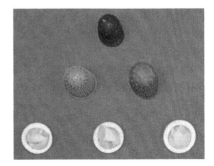

Fig. 2.15 Stripping chalk.

Fig. 2.16 Stripping stone.

Fig. 2.17 Finger covers.

Other products that are required for stripping a coat are:

- Chalk (Fig. 2.15) or powder to get a better grip of the coat.
- Stripping stones (Fig. 2.16) that aid in pulling the coat or scraping out (or carding) the dead undercoat.
- Rubber finger covers (Fig. 2.17), which also help to get a grip on the coat. Even a pair of household rubber gloves will do – just cut the fingers off!

> When hand-stripping keep the skin tight to ensure that the dog is comfortable during the procedure.

The aim of hand-stripping is to remove the dead topcoat and dead undercoat. Always remember to assess the coat to ascertain which hairs need to be removed.

CLIPPERS

Many makes and models of clippers are available (Figs 2.18–2.22) to buy depending on your specific needs. Most professional groomers will choose a clipper with a range of detachable blades.

Clippers are available in single speed, two speed or variable speed; also there are many cordless clippers. It is important when choosing a clipper to feel the weight and comfort of the hold in your hand; what suits one person may not suit another. For the pet market, there are clippers available with a blade with variable depths.

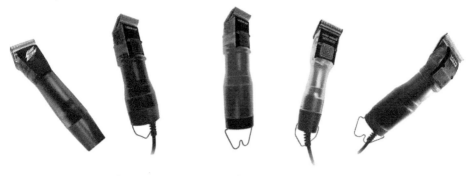

Fig. 2.18 Laube coloured mains and cordless clippers to brighten the salon.

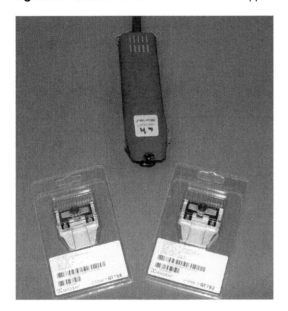

Fig. 2.19 Aesculap mains clippers and blades.

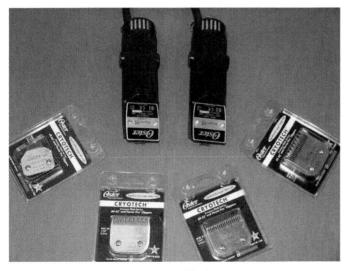

Fig. 2.20 Oster mains clippers and blades.

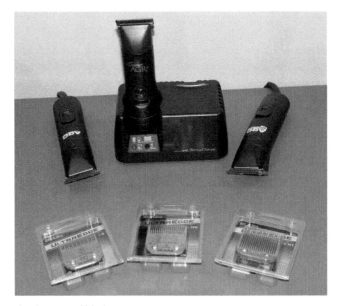

Fig. 2.21 Andis clipper and blades.

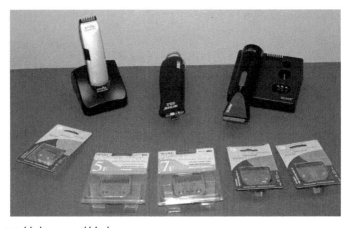

Fig. 2.22 Wahl clipper and blades.

Recommended maintenance of clippers

To maintain your clipper:

- Brush the loose hair away from the moving parts on a regular basis – sometimes you may need to do this during the clipping process if you are working on a very thick coat.

- Professional servicing should be done every six months to one year depending on the use and general care.
- The flex should not be wound around the clipper as this will lead to fractures and failure.
- Clippers should never be dropped, and they should not be stored in a damp environment.

Using clippers

When using a clipper you need to practise manoeuvring your wrist and arm in a wide range of angles. A clipper is used for clipping not only the animal's body but also delicate areas such as ears and groin, so it is important to be flexible and confident while clipping. When holding the clipper try to keep your thumb on top (Fig. 2.23a, b), as this will reduce the strain on the wrist. Keep the hand fairly low down and spread the fingers to balance the weight easily.

Allow the clipper to do the work. Do not force the blade through the coat as this will damage the blade, mark the coat and put pressure on your hand and wrist. Clipping a clean coat will help with this. When dealing with a dirty coat a little pressure may be required. Keep the blade flat on the coat and do not dig the blade in (Fig. 2.24), as this will cause clipping ridges and possible damage to the skin in the more sensitive areas.

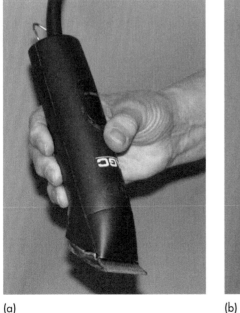
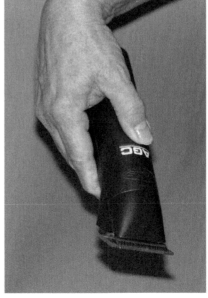

(a) (b)

Fig. 2.23 (a) Holding the clipper with the thumb on top. (b) Clipper hold, still with the thumb on top.

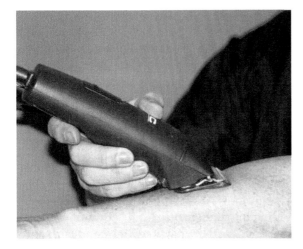

Fig. 2.24 Practise keeping the blade flat.

When clipping the body coat, there is only one straight line and that is the line down the spine. The rest of the clipping follows the 'flow of the coat' and the shape of the dog. When you begin to clip make the line down the spine your first line and then overlap the edges so that no bumps or ridges are left. Be aware of the natural seam at the base of the ears and around the dog's neck where the hair growth changes direction (Figs 2.25 and 2.26). If clipped incorrectly this area can look bald and ruin the overall finish. When working around the rib area, clip in sweeping lines (Figs 2.27 and 2.28) and do not dig in the blade as you will leave lines.

Most body clipping is done following the direction of growth of the coat but the blade can be reversed in some instances, particularly during head trimming. (This

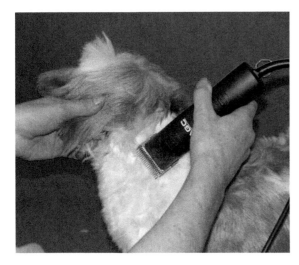

Fig. 2.25 The natural seam at the base of the ear.

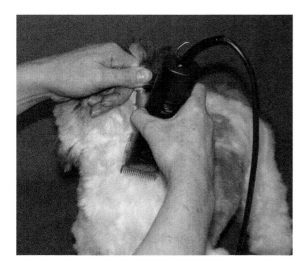

Fig. 2.26 The changing direction of hair growth.

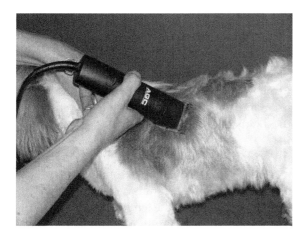

Fig. 2.27 Clip the ribcage area in sweeping lines.

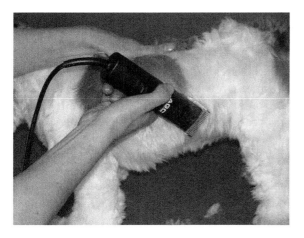

Fig. 2.28 Do not dig in the blade.

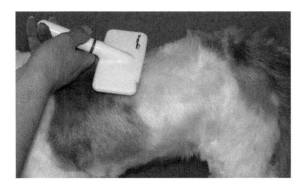

Fig. 2.29 Brush against the growth and re-clip.

is covered in the guidelines for individual breeds, see Chapter 11). Finally, to achieve a good finish with the clipper, lightly brush or comb the coat against the growth (Fig. 2.29) and re-clip. This will ensure a smooth even finish.

BLADES

Blades come in a huge range of sizes depending on the clipper you choose. Detachable blades are commonly used by professional groomers who need to clip a variety of breeds and many styles. Some makes of blades can be interchanged between clippers. However, the best practice is to buy matching clipper and blades to ensure best performance.

Blades must be kept clean, sharp and oiled to gain the best finish on a coat. If blades are used on 'rough' or 'dirty' coats they will become blunt much sooner. Most blades are made of several metal or ceramic components that need to be kept free of hair. If hair gets caught between the teeth, the blade will not clip through the coat. To clean and oil the blades, carefully push the two blades apart and, using a small brush such as a toothbrush or tinting brush, remove any hairs. Blades can be oiled either by drop oil or they can be sprayed with a modern complete care product at regular intervals during working to keep them cool, lubricated and disinfected. These products are easy to use and convenient. Always hold the clipper with the blade on in a downwards direction and spray the specialist product on the working blades in the channels between the two plates of the blade. Stop the clipper after a few seconds and wipe off excess oil with a soft blade cleaning cloth. If you are working on a dirty or matted coat you may need to carry out this process more frequently, as the blade has to work harder.

When using blade washes never leave blades in the wash for more than a few minutes. Always wipe off any residue and dry the blade. To avoid blade pitting or corrosion use drop oil before storing or using the blade. Failure to do this can result in rusting of the blade and may shorten the life span of the blade. Blades will keep a better edge if used on only clean, mat-free dogs.

Blades with broken teeth are dangerous and should never be used, as such blades could cut or graze skin. Blade sharpening and tensioning should always be carried out by a professional. Blades should not be taken apart and self-sharpening may not prove successful. Try not to drop your blades as this will almost certainly knock out the balance and occasionally break the teeth. Always store the blades in a waterproof blade caddy to prevent rusting (Fig. 2.30). Fig. 2.31 shows a range of blade maintenance products.

While clipping you must remain aware of the temperature of the blade as it can get hot very quickly, especially in the summer. If a blade is hot, blunt or dragging

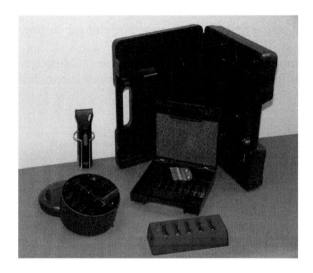

Fig. 2.30 Blade caddies to store blades safely.

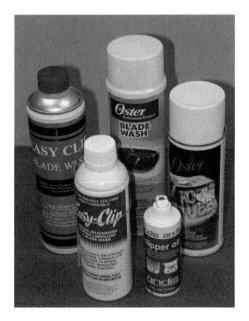

Fig. 2.31 Maintenance products for blades and clippers.

through the coat then 'clipper rash' may occur. Clipper rash, which is a reaction to clipping, results in the dog's skin becoming irritated and sore. It can also be caused by using too fine a blade for the dog's skin. Sometimes you might not be aware of clipper rash developing while you are clipping as the reaction occurs later.

The blade sizes in this book are those present in the most commonly used clippers: Oster, Wahl, Laube and Andis.

COMB ATTACHMENTS

These plastic, snap-on combs clip over a fine blade to give a much longer cutting length. They come in a wide range of sizes and can be useful for quick styling. However, the overall finish is much better with scissors or thinners, although many professional groomers find them invaluable. Their use is more successful on clean, blow dried coats.

SCISSORS

Many sizes and types of scissors are available for grooming. The three main types are: straight, curved and thinning scissors. It is most useful to have a small pair of scissors for delicate areas, i.e. around ears and feet, a long pair for general scissoring and if your dog's coat requires blending or thinning, a pair of thinning scissors.

Scissors are a very individual tool as the size and make you will use will greatly depend on their suitability for *your* hand. All our hands are different and therefore one pair of scissors may feel comfortable and balanced in your hand but not in someone else's. If you are left-handed you may not necessarily need left-handed scissors. Most suppliers will let you handle scissors before you buy any to check that they are right for you. As scissoring is the most important technique to master in grooming it is essential to have what you feel is the best pair of scissors for you.

Scissors come in a range of sizes (Figs 2.32 and 2.33) shapes and prices, but in this instance the more expensive the better. Start your scissors collection with a pair of good all-round scissors, costing approximately £30–40. Then as you become more confident and proficient, build your collection to suit different scissoring needs. A pair of excellent finishing scissors may be expensive but worthwhile.

The metal that scissors are made from and their cutting edge define whether the scissors will be suitable for trimming thick coats or for finer finishing work. Always seek advice before purchasing scissors. Scissors must be cared for and stored correctly. A variety of scissor pouches (Fig. 2.34) are available and only one pair should be stored in one pouch. Scissors should not be stored on their tips in a container as this could damage them.

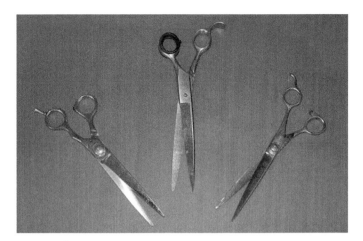

Fig. 2.32 Selection of scissors.

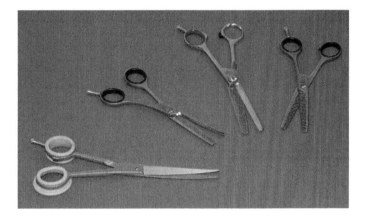

Fig. 2.33 Curved scissors and thinning scissors.

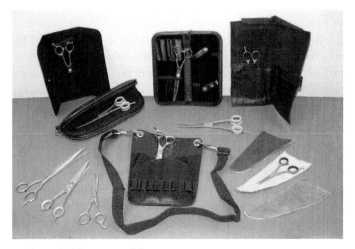

Fig. 2.34 Pouches to hold scissors safely.

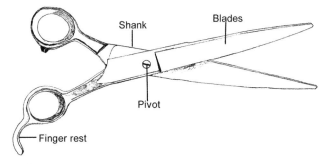

Fig. 2.35 Parts of grooming scissors.

Scissors should never be dropped; if you do drop them get them professionally serviced. Scissors should only be serviced and sharpened by a competent professional. Expensive, top-quality scissors need precision sharpening and servicing. Make sure your technician is competent and understands your requirements. If you are left-handed or have any hand/wrist problems you must tell the technician so they can make sure the servicing accommodates your (the operator's) needs. Oiling and cleaning your scissors is essential to maintain maximum performance. Carefully run a little oil over each blade and around the pivot to keep the parts moving freely. Fig. 2.35 shows the different parts of grooming scissors. Remember to wipe the blade clean before using. Take care! Professional scissors are extremely sharp.

Using scissors

Flexibility and control are vital when using scissors to achieve the preferred smooth, even finish. Balancing and holding the scissors in your hand takes practice but practise you must! Practise holding the scissors as follows:

- Balance them across your hand (Fig. 2.36) and insert the end of the third finger in the finger hole.
- Rest the little finger on the finger rest and balance the middle and index fingers on the shank. The scissors should sit here, quite balanced and steady.
- Insert the end of the thumb into the other finger hole (Fig. 2.37). The thumb does not hold the scissors but it operates them.
- Practise just manoeuvring the thumb to operate the blades.

Scissor exercises

As groomers, we rarely cut in a straight line and thus we need to practise how to use scissors to the best advantage. The following exercises may be of help to you in using your scissors.

Hold your arm straight down by your side (Fig. 2.38), and, while moving the thumb in a scissor action, bring your arm up keeping the shoulder level and the scissors parallel to the floor with the wrist in a relaxed position (Fig. 2.39).

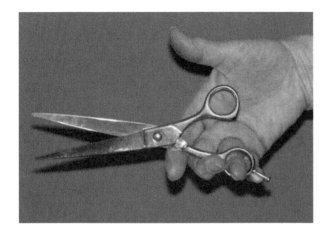

Fig. 2.36 Balance the scissors across your hand.

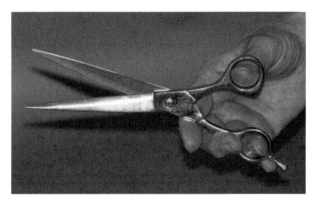

Fig. 2.37 The thumb operates the scissors.

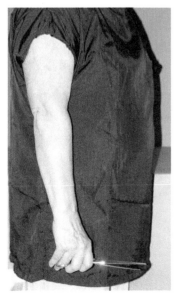

Fig. 2.38 Scissor exercise 1.

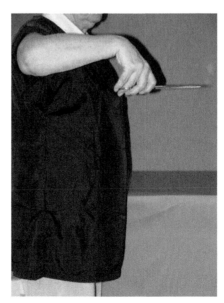

Fig. 2.39 Scissor exercise 2.

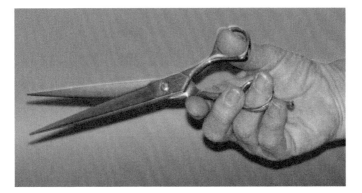

Fig. 2.40 Scissor exercise 3.

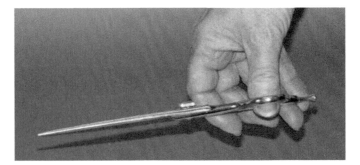

Fig. 2.41 Scissor exercise 4.

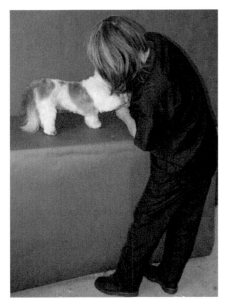

Fig. 2.42 Scissoring stance.

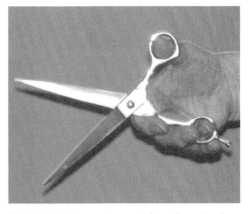

Fig. 2.43 Open scissors wide and use thumb.

Imagine trimming around different shapes, e.g. squares and circles; this will help develop dexterity. Concentrate on keeping the scissors level and even (Figs 2.40 and 2.41). A groomer skilled in the use of scissors trims with the whole of their body and not just the arm. Therefore you must learn to balance from the feet upwards and twist and bend your body (Fig. 2.42) to see the correct trimming line. When one first starts scissoring it is very difficult to stop 'bouncing' the scissors, which results in a choppy finish. To reduce this problem remember to open the scissors wide and move the thumb smoothly (Fig. 2.43).

In conclusion, scissoring is an art form, which takes time to achieve. Don't expect instant results; few people are naturally born to scissor and remember practice makes perfect.

NAIL CLIPPERS

There are basically two types of nail clippers: guillotine or scissors/pliers (Fig. 2.44). The choice is entirely yours.

The clippers come in different sizes to match nail sizes and if you are intending to become a professional groomer, you may require more than one pair. This will be apparent when you come across a nail that has twisted right round (corkscrew nail) and cannot be trimmed with guillotine or blunt pliers. A point-ended nail clipper will be necessary here but great care must be taken to ensure the pad is not damaged. Which ever type of nail clipper you decide on, correct usage is most important (see Chapter 3).

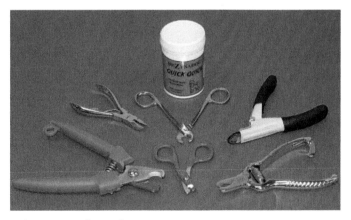

Fig. 2.44 Nail trimmers and coagulant.

EAR CARE

Whether you are a pet owner or professional groomer, ear care is an essential part of the grooming process. The tools required are finger and thumb, and blunt-ended tweezers or artery forceps (Fig. 2.45) to remove any hair growing in the ear canal. (Fig. 2.46) (see Chapter 3 for the ear care procedure). Powders can be used

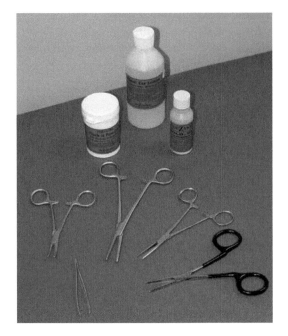

Fig. 2.45 Ear cleaning products and tools.

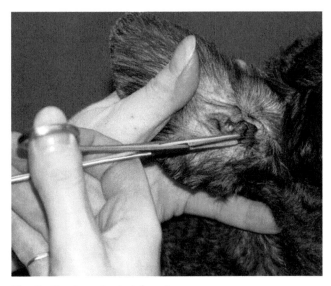

Fig. 2.46 Removing hair from the ear.

to help get a better grip on the hair but care must be taken not to use these excessively as they could block the ears.

TOOLBOX

It is most useful to keep all your tools and equipment together for easy access and organisation. A purpose-made toolbox can be used (Fig. 2.47) or you could investigate your local do-it-yourself store for a cheaper option. Grooming trolleys may also be useful in the salon.

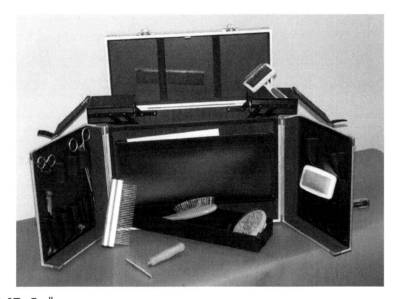

Fig. 2.47 Toolbox.

RESTRAINTS

It is important while working on a dog to have control, whether in a pet, show or professional situation. There are various methods of restraint from neck collars to belly straps and muzzles (Fig. 2.48). However, the best method of control is to build a confident relationship with the dog.

When using restraints, consider the dog's temperament, age and health condition. If tethering a dog never leave it unattended on a workbench or table as the dog could try to jump and thus hang itself.

Professional groomers most commonly use nylon restraints, as they dry easily if they get wet and can be cut through quickly if the dog twists itself around it. Muzzles must be used with respect for the dog. Most dogs that bite have a genuine reason to do so, e.g. they are nervous or in pain. There are very few evil dogs out there!

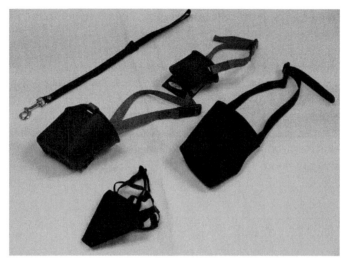

Fig. 2.48 Restraints and muzzles.

A Halti can also be used as a restraint but one person will be required to hold the head end, so they are not much use if you are working on your own.

GROOMING TABLES AND WORK STOOLS

Choosing a grooming table is a most important point to consider. What do you need from it? There are basically three types of table:

- Electric (Figs 2.49 and 2.50)
- Hydraulic
- Static (Fig. 2.51)

If you are grooming only your own dog then a static table would be the cheapest option for you. However, if you are considering a career in grooming then an adjustable height table (Fig. 2.50) will suit your needs better. The table must be steadfast and have a non-slip surface to ensure the dog's safety and comfort. Many tables come with a holding frame, which is essential for the professional groomer.

Grooming stools (Fig. 2.52) can be of great benefit. You will usually stand to trim your dog but just resting on a stool can help alleviate the pressure in your back and legs.

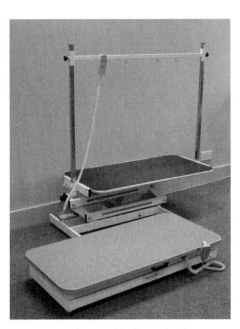

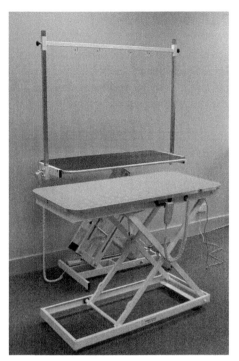

Fig. 2.49 Electric table (lowest level).

Fig. 2.50 Electric table (highest level).

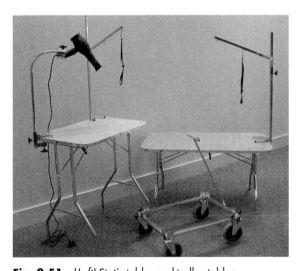

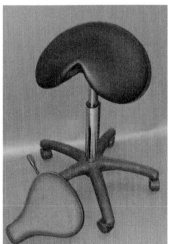

Fig. 2.51 (*Left*) Static tables and trolley tables.
Fig. 2.52 (*Right*) Mobile stool with a choice of seats.

OILING EQUIPMENT

Equipment of all types should be kept cleaned and oiled or greased according to the manufacturer's recommendations. In a salon situation, rusting can be a serious issue. A dehumidifier is a good investment and can lengthen the life span of equipment.

STERILISATION

Ultraviolet (UV) sterilisation is by far the preferred method. It is good practice to sterilise each item after every dog, particularly if an animal gives the groomer any reason to suspect that something contagious could be present. At the very least, equipment such as brushes, combs, forceps and any other direct-contact equipment should be sterilised at the end of each working day. If spray-on sterilisation fluid is used the equipment must be dried completely and then oiled to prevent rusting.

FINISHING TOUCHES

Many pet owners or professional groomers may enjoy adding bows or perfumes as finishing touches (Fig. 2.53) to their neat and clean dog. There are many accessories readily available to buy. A patterned collar and lead could be all you need, or in extreme cases tiaras, t-shirts or even bandanas. Whatever finishing touches you choose, try to remember that the dog is a dog and not a doll for dressing up.

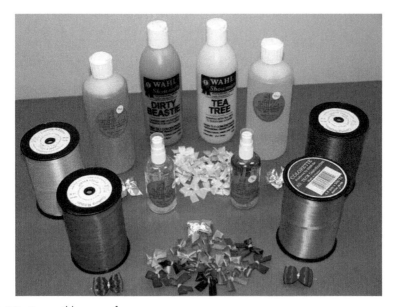

Fig. 2.53 Bows, ribbons, perfumes.

Pre-grooming and General Care

3

Without being aware of it, every time you handle an animal you are assessing its health status. A healthy animal is alert, ready to exercise, constantly observing humans in its environment and generally is a creature of habit. Deviation from normal habits and character may be cause for concern. A healthy animal will not have any of the following:

- Unpleasant or new odours
- Discharge from the mouth, nose, eyes, ears, body or uro-genital areas
- Loss of appetite (Fig. 3.1)
- Increase in thirst and frequency of urination
- Diarrhoea or vomiting
- Difficulty in moving
- Breathing problems
- Unwillingness to exercise (Fig. 3.2)

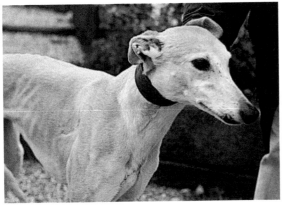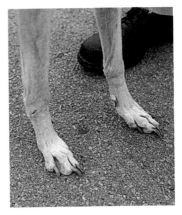

Fig. 3.1 (*Left*) A Greyhound with a loose tooth affecting its ability to eat.
Fig. 3.2 (*Right*) A Greyhound with long toe nails because of inability to exercise.

Outside their home environment many animals feel stressed. Signs of anxiety and stress in an animal include:

- Excessive salivation
- Shivering
- Aggression/fear
- Rapid breathing/panting
- Rapid pulse and heart rate
- Pale mucous membranes

If an animal has a medical condition it may respond in one or more of the above listed ways when in strange surroundings. Always take this into account when handling an animal, and if you have any concerns, report them to the owner.

Grooming will be a daily and/or a weekly event for the owner depending on the type of coat of the dog or cat. A cat that moults or sheds coat hair in spring needs careful grooming assistance from its owner, especially if it has a long or semi-long coat. Otherwise it can swallow a lot of loose hair while self grooming, resulting in a hair ball, which may then require veterinary attention.

Grooming provides an opportunity to check and assist in the maintenance of an animal's health. In the grooming salon a systematic approach to the animal as a whole should be employed as described in the following sections.

EYES

The eyes should be bright and free of any discharge. The third eyelid, also known as the nictitating membrane, should be in the normal position (i.e. below the lower lid, just visible in the inner corner of the eye). Ideally, the eyes should be cleaned before grooming. Clean away any debris or dried tears as follows:

- Gently supporting the animal's head and with a piece of cotton wool moistened with warm water wipe from the inner corner of the eye, down over the upper lid to the nose (Fig. 3.3).

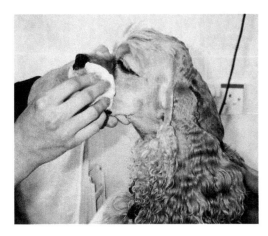

Fig. 3.3 Support the head while wiping the eyes.

- Turn the cotton wool after completing the movement, to prevent replacing the dry material from the inner corner of the eye. Repeat the movement as required.
- Finally, wipe the whole eyelid area in the direction of the coat hair.
- Dispose of the cotton wool used for the first eye and start again on the other eye with a new piece of moistened cotton wool.

EARS

The ears should be free of wax and hair. They should be a dull pink colour and without odour. Check for signs of discomfort, smell or reluctance by the animal when examining the ear flap (Fig. 3.4) as described below.

- Lift the ear flap gently to open the ear canal.
- Moisten a piece of cotton wool with warm water and wipe away any ear wax or dirt from the ear canal (Fig. 3.5). This may require more than one piece of cotton wool.
- Repeat this to include the outer cartilaginous section of the ear flap, gently wiping between the cartilage valleys. Wipe dry.
- If required, pluck any long hair from inside the ear canal using your fingers only. Take hold of the ear flap, lift it up and lay it flat on the dog's head. This protects the ear canal by closing it and at the same time gives a clear view of the outer ear.
- Pull only a few hairs at a time with quick firm movements (Fig. 3.6).

Cotton buds (if being used) should not be put into the ear canal. If the animal moves, the ear drum can get damaged. Buds should only be used on the external ear to wipe any wax that has shaken free from the canal.

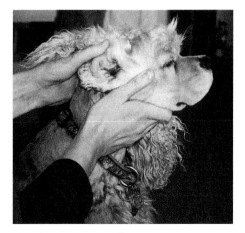 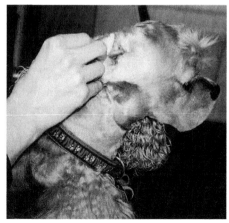

Fig. 3.4 Examining the ear.   **Fig. 3.5** Clean the outer ear canal of wax.

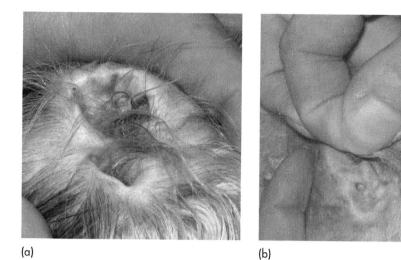

(a)   (b)

Fig. 3.6   (a) Hair in the ear. (b) Plucking hair from the ear canal and outer ear.

Hair can trap the wax, which head shaking would normally throw to the outer ear. The wax attracts parasites such as the ear mite (*Otodectes*), which could lead to infection (see Chapter 8).

Use powders **only** around the outer ear, because powder if moistened can form a paste, which can move down and block the ear canal.

MOUTH

Check that the gums and tongue are pink (except in breeds with pigmented tongues and gums, e.g. Chow Chow) or partly pink with pigmented areas. Gums should be well defined around each tooth, with no food or other materials sticking to them (Fig. 3.7). The gums should not be sore (gingivitis) and there should be no unusual odours in the breath.

Check that the teeth are not damaged and are a normal white colour with no tartar deposits. Regular use of pet toothpaste while cleaning the teeth, if the animal allows, can help prevent build-up of tartar on the teeth. Gently brush the teeth using the toothpaste, toothbrush or, alternatively, a finger brush on the outer surfaces of lower and upper teeth. Removal of tartar should be done by a veterinary surgeon. Record and report any observations to the owner.

- Before brushing teeth **assess the animal's temperament**.
- Never forget that the teeth of dogs and cats are designed for killing prey and tearing flesh!
- Start teeth cleaning in an animal when it is young to make it a part of the animal's routine early in life.

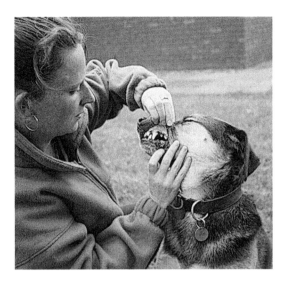

Fig. 3.7 Examining the gums and teeth.

FACIAL CARE

Special care is required for breeds with facial skin folds, e.g. Shar Pei or Pug. To prevent skin inflammation and infections in skin folds it is essential to keep the wrinkles clean and dry as described below.

- Wipe the skin with cotton wool moistened in warm water.
- Wipe the whole face in the same direction as the lie of the coat hair, replacing the cotton wool with clean ones as necessary (Fig. 3.8).
- Dry each fold area in turn.

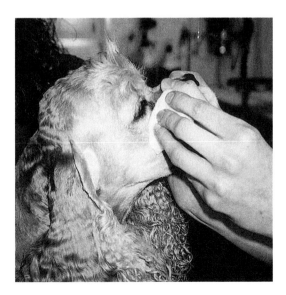

Fig. 3.8 Wipe the face with moistened cotton wool.

- While cleaning, check each fold for signs of redness and record and report if any.
- Check the rest of the face for parasites, lumps/bumps and any kind of skin change.

NAIL AND CLAW CARE

The feet should be clean around the nail bed, with nails just in contact with the ground. Any excess hair should be cut short between the pads and nails to prevent mats and grass seed barbs penetrating the skin and causing inflammation or infection.

Nails that are pigmented black tend to have longer nail beds, so beware of cutting off too much. The area inside the nail, which cannot be seen, is called the nail bed, or quick, and contains the blood supply and nerves.

Dogs have four toes on each foot, and each toe has a pad and a nail. In addition, nails may be present slightly higher on the inside of the leg. These are called dew nails. Some breeds have extra or supernumerary toes, e.g. Pyrenean Mountain and Newfoundland. Active, healthy dogs do not need frequent nail clipping. The nails will wear naturally with everyday use to remain just clear of, or just touching, the ground when standing normally. An exception may be the dew nail, which can grow into the nail bed if left unchecked (although they tend to be slow growing in most breeds).

Cats have five toes on the front feet and four toes on the back feet. Each toe has a claw, which is kept retracted most of the time. Occasionally, a cat's claws will need attention, particularly in older animals.

The procedure for clipping nails in dogs and claws in cats is as follows:

- Restrain and reassure the animal before and during the procedure.
- Spread each foot and inspect the area between the toes.
- Select the correct nail clipper (Fig. 3.9).
- Inspect each foot, identifying the nails or claws that need attention. Squeeze each toe gently between the thumb and forefinger placed above and below the toe, respectively, to extend the nail or claw.
- Locate the 'quick' (nerve and blood supply).
- Cut below the quick (only if required), removing only the pointed tip of the nail or claw (Fig. 3.10).
- Smooth any rough edges with a nail file.

Have a styptic pencil or other coagulant agent at hand to stop any bleeding just in case the quick is cut.

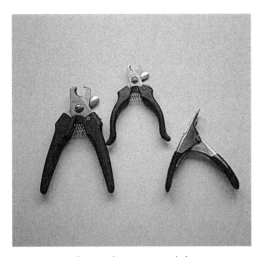

Fig. 3.9 Selecting the correct nail clipper.

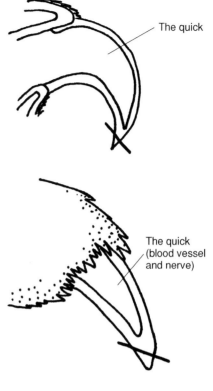

The quick

The quick
(blood vessel
and nerve)

Fig. 3.10 (*Right*) Nail clipping: cut below
the 'quick' so that only the pointed tip of the nail
is removed.

ANAL GLANDS

The anal glands are situated on either side of the anus, positioned at 4 o'clock and
8 o'clock with their ducts leading to openings at the anal rim (Fig. 3.11). The secretion of the anal glands has an unpleasant smell, and it is thought the animal uses it
as a pheromone when marking territory. Occasionally a duct can get blocked and
the anal sac will need to be emptied. If a dog is seen licking the anal region or
drags its rear along the ground, this may mean that the glands are causing some
irritation and discomfort and need to be emptied.

If on examination prior to emptying the glands, they appear red, swollen or
painful, do not empty but recommend the owner to seek veterinary advice. While
emptying the glands, it is helpful if one person concentrates on restraining the
animal, allowing the second person to empty the glands safely. The procedure for
emptying anal glands is as follows:

- Wear gloves. (This is important for protection of the person who will empty the
  glands.)
- Place a pad of cotton wool across the palm of one hand.
- Raise the dog's tail with the other hand (Fig. 3.12).
- Hold the pad at the anal region.

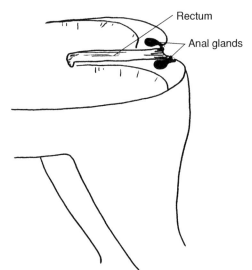

Rectum

Anal glands

Fig. 3.11 Diagram illustrating the position of the anal glands.

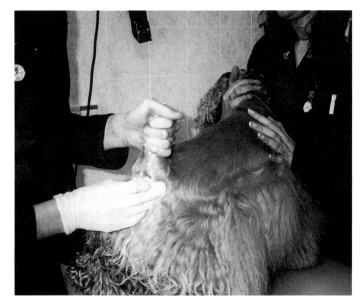

Fig. 3.12 The handler restrains the dog and the operator holds the tail while emptying the anal glands.

- With the middle finger and thumb placed on either side of the anus squeeze, pushing gently towards the anus. At the same time, squeeze upwards with the other fingers partly behind the anal gland to empty the contents.
- Clean the anal region and dispose of contaminated cotton wool.

During the pre-grooming examination of the animal described above it is useful to note any changes such as:

- Loss of hair and location.
- Changes in coat colour.
- A pot-bellied appearance due to changes in muscle and skin tone.

In some diseases, the skin can appear thin, with surface blood vessels clearly visible. The skin may bruise easily with the appearance of small bleeding points (pin points) under the skin surface (haematomas). Loss of hair (alopecia) may range from slight thinning to complete loss on whole sections of the animal's body. Record and report to the owner if any alteration is noticed.

CAUSES OF HAIR LOSS

- **Feline symmetrical alopecia**: This is also known as feline hormonal alopecia. It may be seen in neutered cats with hair loss initially around the anal region and then in the abdominal and groin areas.
- **Sertoli cell tumour**: This is a testicular tumour seen in middle-aged and old dogs. The hair loss is seen bilaterally in the flanks, around the anal region, abdomen, and groin area.
- **External parasites**: Hair loss associated with parasites is usually seen in a localised area, where the animal has been scratching itself, e.g. with surface/subsurface parasites (fleas, lice and mites). Hair loss due to ringworm (dermatophytes or fungal spores) infection occurs in circular areas. The affected area has a red, raised circular margin.
- **Calluses**: These are located, in particular, on the elbows and hock region of heavy dogs, and are caused by excessive pressure on the area from a hard surface. Hair loss and thickening of the skin are seen.

LUMPS AND BUMPS

A tumour is an abnormal tissue swelling that occurs when growth and division of the cells exceeds that of the surrounding normal tissue cells. Tumours can appear anywhere in or on the body. Some are very slow growing and are usually independent or movable relative to the neighbouring tissues. Others may grow quickly or slowly, do not have an independent shape and invade the local tissues as well.

Record and report to the owner if any have appeared since the last visit to the grooming salon.

Skin tumours

- **Warts** (papilloma): These are tumours of the epithelial cells, seen in both dogs and cats, and are often located on the lips, mouth, eyelids, and ears.
- **Lipomas**: These are tumours of surface fat cells, seen in older or obese animals. They can be moved freely when the skin over them is lifted.

- **Cysts**: These are swellings which contain fluid (not blood or pus). The commonest form occurs when a secretory skin gland gets blocked, thus preventing escape of the fluid through its duct. Cysts may be **sebaceous** cysts or **interdigital** cysts. Sebaceous cysts are seen in older animals and are situated within the skin. The contents are sticky and viscous, and as a consequence the cyst feels quite firm. Interdigital cysts are seen between the toes. Many contain a foreign body, e.g. grass seed.

Hernias

A hernia is seen as a lump in the skin in certain locations on the body when an organ or tissue protrudes through an opening in the body wall. They do not cause any pain to the animal except when the organ or tissue becomes strangulated. Hernias are described by their location:

- **Inguinal hernia**: This occurs in the groin and may contain uterus, intestines or bladder. It is seen as a swelling in the groin, extending towards the vulva/anal region.
- **Umbilical hernia**: This occurs at the navel and is usually seen in young animals. As the animal grows it is less likely to allow tissues to protrude. However, if the hernia is large enough to allow protrusion as the animal grows, the risk of entrapment of tissue and strangulation of the blood supply is increased.

Animals coming into the grooming salon may have had surgery in the past. It is useful to have records of any extensive tumour removal, and corrective surgery such as aural resection (surgery of the ear), urethral opening and laparotomy (mid-line scar visible on the abdomen). It is often easier to detect changes in an animal in the grooming salon with reference to records because of the time interval between grooming sessions. Many changes will be insignificant; however, some may give cause for concern and need veterinary investigation. In spite of records, it is important to always run through a superficial examination to update information and avoid areas of the skin surface that may be sore or painful. Examples of changes that may be seen include:

- Weight changes
- Appearance of lumps and bumps or increase in size of existing ones
- Pain on handling
- Skin or hair changes
- Breathing difficulties
- Obesity

Good practice in the grooming parlour that helps the animal and its owner includes:

- Observation
- Recording
- Reporting

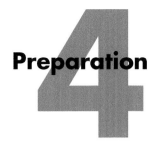

Preparation

DOGS

Handling

Before any grooming procedure is carried out, it is important to understand the correct way to handle a dog. Grooming should be a pleasurable and rewarding experience for both dog and groomer, and should not be seen as some torturous experience that the dog begins to dread! Body language is the key: the ability to understand basic dog signs will make you a better handler.

Remember the five freedoms when working with dogs and cats:

- Freedom from fear and stress
- Freedom from pain, injury and disease
- Freedom from hunger and thirst
- Freedom from discomfort
- Freedom to express most normal behaviour

In the salon the third freedom (freedom from hunger and thirst) may not apply, except water must be available if required.

Introducing a dog to grooming and handling

A dog's natural instinct is to protect its feet and belly. Dogs need good feet to chase and catch prey to survive and an open belly usually means death. It is therefore advisable to begin grooming other areas of the dog first. If any unfamiliar animal goes for, or touches these areas, the dog will assume it is being attacked.

In the case of pets, handling the dog all over its body on a daily basis of small ten-minute sessions will increase its trust in you. Introduction of grooming tools should be done with a steady approach and consideration. Figs 4.1–4.4 show how to introduce a puppy to grooming. If the puppy tries to bite or scream, pause, but continue to hold the puppy gently but firmly. If you immediately release the puppy when it screams it will learn that this is the way to stop the process. This

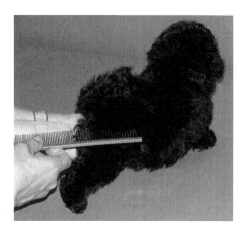

Fig. 4.1 Introducing a puppy to grooming: begin with the easy areas.

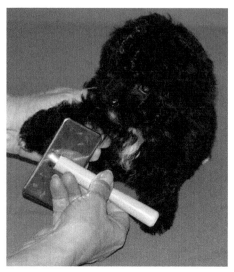

Fig. 4.2 Gradually work towards the problem areas.

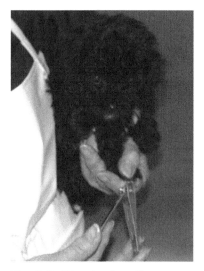

Fig. 4.3 Trimming the nails.

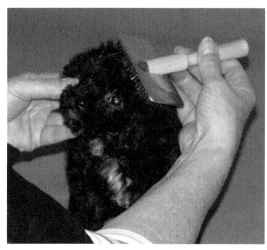

Fig. 4.4 Brushing the head.

could lead to the puppy becoming impossible to groom when an adult dog. Stay calm during the process and hold the feet or beard – the screaming can continue for a while! Begin grooming again in an easier area and gradually work towards the problem area soothing and praising the dog when it is still and accepting the process.

Human–dog interaction

Dogs' behaviour towards people moves between three states:

- From being friendly and enjoying interactions
- Through to arousal when ready to defend themselves if need be
- To fearful, seeking to avoid interaction

Friendly dogs (Fig. 4.5) will be calm with soft eye contact and will move easily. The tail is usually carried at medium height and often with a relaxed wag. If you greet them, the tail will drop slightly and they may raise a paw. The ears are relaxed and carried low and they may seek contact with you by leaning on you or towards your stroking hand.

Fearful dogs (Fig. 4.6a, b) will seek to move away from the object of fear, in this case the groomer or other dogs. The tail is carried low, often tucked hard between the legs. Early signs of fear include lip licking and grimacing (showing teeth with the lips pulled back) (Fig. 4.7). The ears are usually flat against the head with a low or crouching body posture and the dog avoids eye contact. Its eyes will glance around and hackles may be raised. Watch for slow, stiff movements and air sniffing. Barking will be non-rhythmic and the anal glands may empty or the dog may urinate.

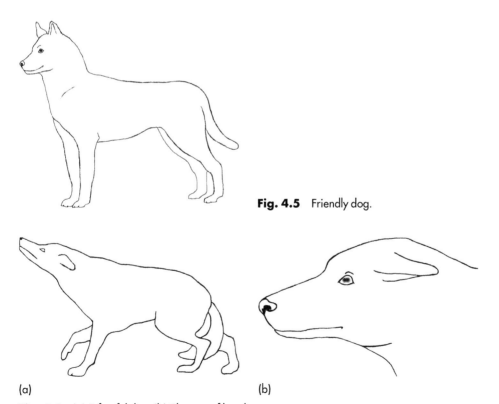

Fig. 4.5 Friendly dog.

(a)   (b)

Fig. 4.6 (a) A fearful dog. (b) Close up of head.

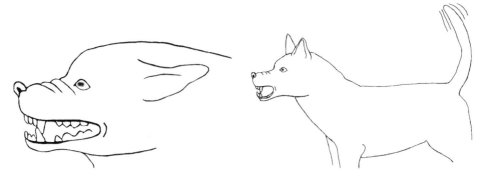

Fig. 4.7 (*left*) Fearful dog – head with teeth showing.   **Fig. 4.8** (*Right*) Aroused dog.

Aroused dogs (Fig. 4.8) are ready to defend themselves. Their sniffing will be intrusive – 'full on'. Eye contact will be long and hard. They will move stiffly with high tail carriage. There may be a stiff wag, typically just the tip. If you move too close they may react and jump. Growling will be low and deep with bared teeth and stiff, forward ear carriage. Other behaviours that may be seen are mounting, flirting, licking genitals of other dogs and rapid vertical tail wagging (inappropriate sexual posturing).

Both fearful and aroused dogs have dilated pupils – if you can get close enough to see! There are a lot of grey areas with these behaviours. A fearful dog may want to be social but lack the confidence to interact. Dogs may show a combination of signals from all three stages on the behaviour scale described above. You also have to bear in mind that breed type, age, sex and history will also have an effect. Your observations will help you to interact with them and increase their confidence.

Signs of stress include yawning, lip licking, ears carried back and close to the head, dilated pupils, occasional grumbling, crouched posture, urination, tight muzzle panting with the corners drawn back and large dilated pupils.

Beware of common misconceptions:

- Tail wagging does not always mean friendliness.
- Raised hackles does not always mean aggression.
- Jumping up does not always mean friendliness or dominance.
- Sitting on your lap is not always a sign of friendliness.
- Rolling on the back is not always a sign of submission.

Avoid thinking in terms of dominance with dogs. Truly dominant dogs are rare. Pushy, confident and bullying dogs are common. These can be considered as dogs with more opinions about certain things than other dogs. They are also more likely to react if asked or made to do something that they don't want to do or don't like.

In the salon

Remember safety of staff and yourself and take precautions with very fearful or reactive dogs. A dog in a holding enclosure may sometimes become protective of its environment and therefore it is a good idea to keep a lead on the dog, with its end outside the crate to avoid you risking being bitten. Take hold of the lead first then encourage the dog to come out. Avoid direct eye-to-eye contact with new dogs until you have assessed their body signals.

Experience in handling can only be built up with time, but a confident handling technique will enable a better relationship between you and the dog. If you show nervousness in your approach the dog will react to this.

Dog–dog interaction

Awareness of dog-to-dog interaction is important. The same signals will be given to other dogs in the salon.

- Avoid putting reactive dogs in places where there will be a lot of passing activity by people or dogs.
- Timid, fearful dogs should be kept near quiet but friendly dogs and away from busy areas.

Always be aware of the dogs in your care to avoid any conflicts. Place yourself between two dogs if they need to pass by each other.

Grooming out

Whatever the coat type, with the exception of smooth coats, the grooming out procedure is the same. The choice of equipment will vary, depending on whether the dog being groomed is a pet or a show dog. Before any finishing procedures can be carried out it is important that the dog's coat is clean and free of knots.

> Always assess the coat for condition, type and skin problems before beginning grooming.

With the exception of hand-stripping, it is always preferable to trim a freshly bathed coat. Wire coats must be hand-stripped before bathing as bathing softens the texture of the coat, which makes stripping more difficult.

Dogs may not require brushing before the bath if their coat is maintained regularly between trims. In fact sometimes it is much easier to remove dead undercoat and knots after bathing, using the correct drying techniques. A good general-purpose brush for pet and commercial use is the slicker brush, and this brush and a medium-width toothcomb should suffice for grooming out. However, if the coat is matted then a de-matter, scissors or clippers may be necessary (Fig. 4.9).

For show dogs, particularly for silk coats and some double coats, a pin or bristle brush should be used to prevent breakage of the coat. These brushes will not

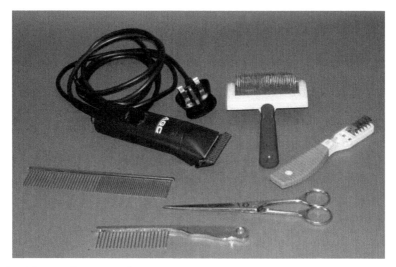

Fig. 4.9 Selection of equipment for grooming out.

remove mats, and if the coat gets into a matted state then a slicker brush may have to be used. However, in this book we are not dealing with show grooming and we therefore suggest that you seek advice from breed specialists for specific show grooming techniques.

Whichever process you are carrying out, whether it is grooming out, bathing, drying or trimming, it is always best to work to a routine. This will ensure that all the areas of the dog are dealt with.

Start at the foot of one of the rear legs of the dog (Fig. 4.10), lift the coat up and brush from the bottom of the coat outwards. Try to keep tension on the skin, as this will prevent unnecessary pulling. Ensure that you are brushing to the skin and not just skimming over the top – be aware of brush burn.

Work your way up the leg and into the body (Fig. 4.11) and continue along the side of the body and into the shoulder (Fig. 4.12).

Move on to the foot of the front leg and meet up with the shoulder (Fig. 4.13). Remember the armpit! Brush out the chest and throat (Fig. 4.14) working your way round to the back of the neck (Fig. 4.15). Brush one side of the head, the ear and beard and then do the other side (Fig. 4.16).

Repeat the whole process on the other side of the dog, finishing by brushing the tail (Fig. 4.17).

Comb through the coat only when the brushing is complete. A comb will not glide through a dirty coat but will help you to find any major knots that you may have missed before. Different coat types require different combing techniques.

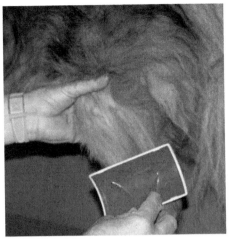

Fig. 4.10 Start at the foot of one of the rear legs.

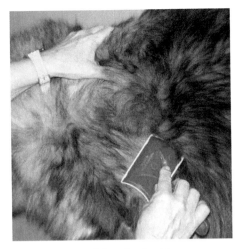

Fig. 4.13 Work into the shoulder.

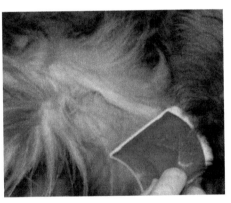

Fig. 4.11 Work up the leg to the body.

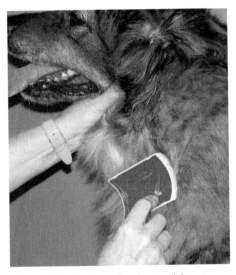

Fig. 4.14 Brush out the chest and throat.

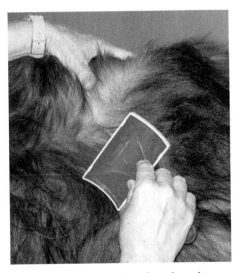

Fig. 4.12 Continue along the side and into the shoulder.

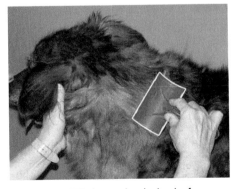

Fig. 4.15 Work round to the back of the neck.

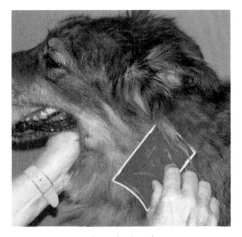

Fig. 4.16 Brushing the head.

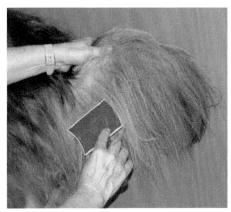

Fig. 4.17 Brushing the tail.

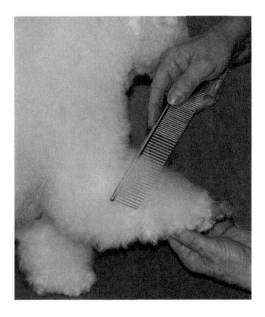

Fig. 4.18 A wool coat should be combed from the base.

A wool coat should be combed from the base and tossed outwards (Fig. 4.18). A silk coat should be combed straight down from root to tip (Fig. 4.19).

Matted coats

A mat is formed by the dead undercoat clumping together or by a longer coat becoming twisted. If a matted coat becomes wet then the mats will tighten and almost become solid. Figs 4.20 and 4.21 show how mats can tighten together.

A de-matter should be used in conjunction with a brush. Brush the knot or mat to open it first (Fig. 4.22) and then carefully use the de-matter (Fig. 4.23) to break open the coat. Brush again to release the mat. Do not pull the mat out with the

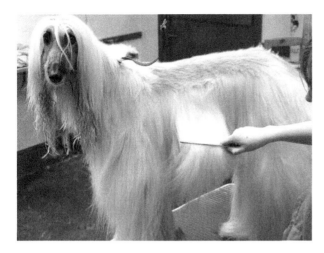

Fig. 4.19 Silk coat – combed straight down from the root to tip.

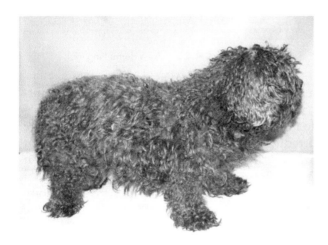

Fig. 4.20 A totally matted coat.

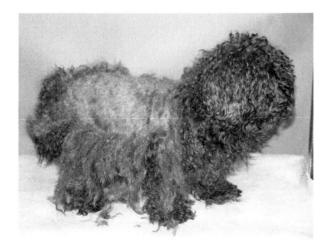

Fig. 4.21 A partly clipped matted coat.

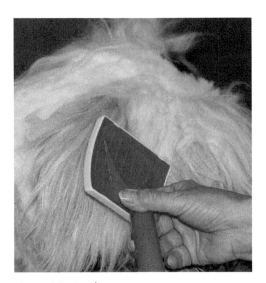

Fig. 4.22 Brush mat open.

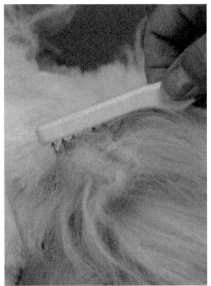

Fig. 4.23 Use a de-matting tool.

de-matter as this will be most uncomfortable for the dog. Keep the skin taut during this procedure.

Unfortunately the use of a de-matter does result in loss of coat, as the teeth are blades. Use of a brush would reduce the loss, and our experience shows that brushes can remove most mats if used correctly. If a coat is so severely matted that grooming out would cause the dog distress and discomfort, removal of the coat with clippers or scissors will be necessary. When using scissors on matted, knotty coats remember not to use your best pair as working through knots will blunt the cutting edge. **Always cut through the knots away from the skin** (Fig. 4.24).

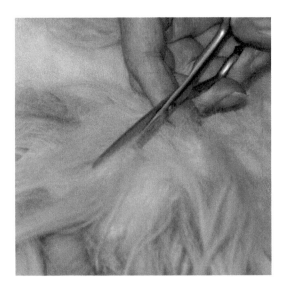

Fig. 4.24 Cut knots away from skin.

After this, brush the two split areas or use a de-matter to separate further. When using a clipper to remove mats remember that the machine has to work hard so you may need to oil the blades as you are working. The most important point to remember is not to force the blade through the knots but to work underneath them. (Figs 4.25–4.27). **Be very aware of the temperature of the blade to avoid clipper rash**.

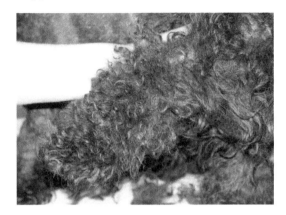

Fig. 4.25 Mat that needs to be removed with a clipper.

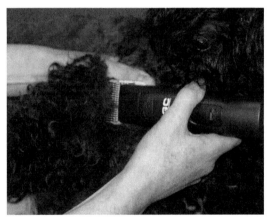

Fig. 4.26 Work underneath the mat.

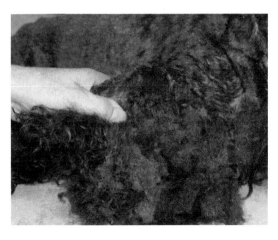

Fig. 4.27 Work with care around the armpit.

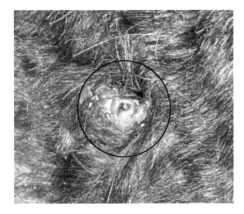

Fig. 4.28 Beware of hidden bumps and lumps.

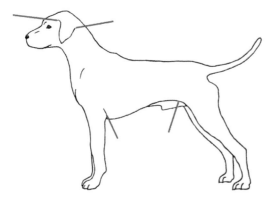

Fig. 4.29 Danger areas.

The selection of blade size depends on the severity of matting but generally a 7F for body and a no. 10 for finer areas would work well. Be careful of loose skin, lumps and bumps (Fig. 4.28) entangled in the mat. Danger areas are armpits, flanks and ears. (Fig. 4.29).

If you are working in a commercial salon, always inform the owner of a dog with a matted coat before any clipping off is carried out. Explain the reason why this is necessary and that the dog will be less stressed with this option. Suggest a regular grooming programme to prevent re-occurrence. Always try to leave the dog a little dignity, i.e. a little hair on the tail if a long tail and a little around the eyes (Fig. 4.30).

There are some breeds where it is totally unacceptable to clip off, such as Rough Collie (Pa–Dc1), Samoyed (Pa–Dc1) and Chow Chow (Ut–Dc1). Note that these breeds are all heavy double coated, and a clip off not only looks dreadful but is also totally degrading for the dog. Thus it should be avoided at all costs unless the vet advises it for medical reasons. A slicker brush, a wide toothcomb and a blaster will all help to remove dead undercoat.

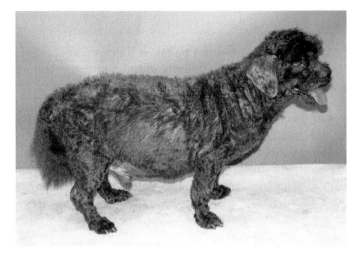

Fig. 4.30 A completed clip off.

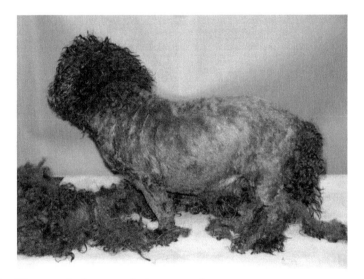

Fig. 4.31 Clip excess body coat and scissor excess leg coat.

Rough trimming

Some dogs may require some coat removal prior to bathing; usually we will only suggest this if the coat is quite over-grown. Clip the excess body coat according to the breed styling required and carefully scissor excessive leg coat (Fig. 4.31). Remember not to go too short as the coat is dirty and will not be finished correctly.

CATS

Cat grooming is a job that should not be taken lightly. Cats can be difficult to groom if they are not accustomed to it. Early introduction to grooming tools and equipment will help to ease the task and get the cat used to procedures and routines. Figs 4.32–4.35 show some cats being groomed.

A cat's temperament is totally different from that of a dog. One cannot communicate with cats in the same way as with dogs or as easily and cats will not respond to commands. A cat cannot be fastened by a lead so it may be advantageous to have a second person to help in difficult areas such as armpits and groins. Cats do not like loud or sudden noises, so a quiet area is best when grooming a cat.

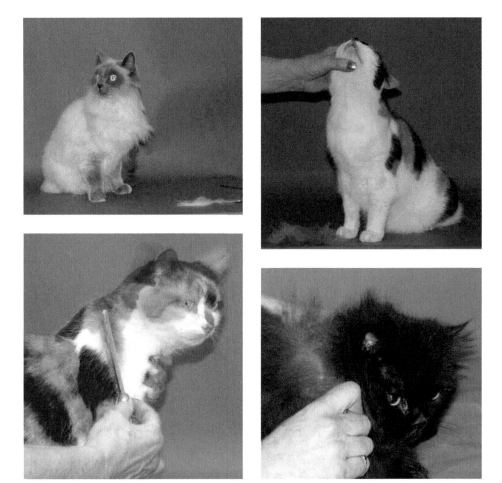

Figs. 4.32–4.35 Cats being groomed.

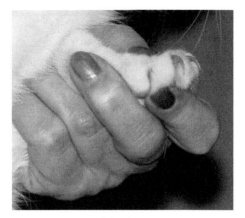

Fig. 4.36 Extend the claw.

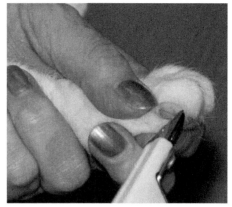

Fig. 4.37 Clip the claw.

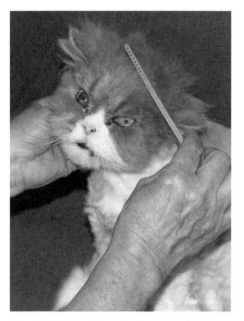
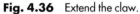

Fig. 4.38 Use the comb to groom all areas.

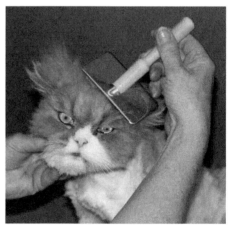

Fig. 4.39 Use the brush on legs and head.

Cutting the cat's nails first can be an advantage. Hold the foot firmly putting your finger on the underside of the pad to extend the claw (Fig. 4.36) and cut the nail (Fig. 4.37) taking care to avoid the quick (see Chapter 3). Use a medium-length toothcomb and a soft slicker brush and pin or bristle brush to finish. Use the comb to groom all areas of the cat (Fig. 4.38). The slicker can be used on the legs and head on thick long coated breeds (Fig. 4.39).

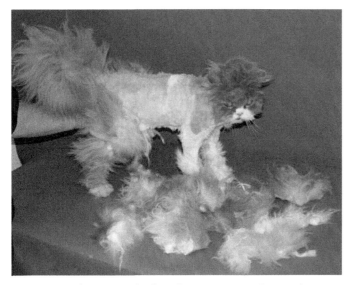

Fig. 4.40 Clipping may be the only option in severely matted cases.

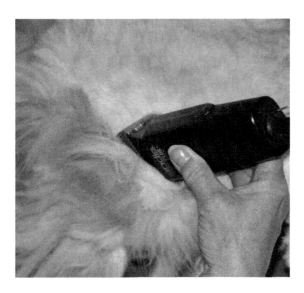

Fig. 4.41 Use a fine blade on delicate areas.

If the cat is knotty be very careful not to split the skin if using a de-matter. In the most severe cases, clipping off may be the only option (Fig. 4.40). **Remember that a cat's skin is very thin and tears or cuts easily**.

Use a fine blade for delicate areas such as armpits and groin. A fine blade would be usually a size 10–50 depending on the severity of matting (Fig. 4.41).

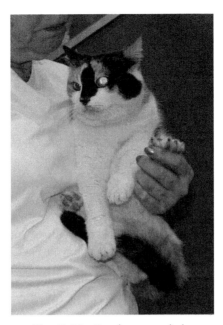

Fig. 4.42 Rest the cat regularly.

Remember to check the blade frequently so that it does not get hot. Be aware of your limitations and when it is advisable to refer the cat to the vet for sedated grooming.

In all instances of cat grooming, work for short periods of time, guided by the cat's temperament, and allow the cat to rest in between each session (Fig. 4.42).

And so to the bath!

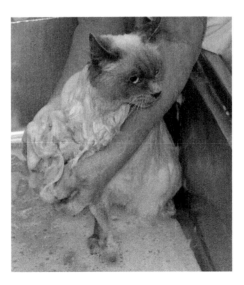

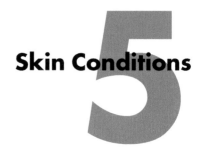

Skin Conditions

The coat of a dog or cat is often its most striking feature, but it is the skin beneath the coat that is the more complex structure of the two. The skin is the largest organ of the body, and it has a number of functions that are essential for the well-being of the animal. The skin forms a continuous layer over the body, and it is also continuous with the mucous membranes of the mouth, nose and genital openings.

STRUCTURE OF THE SKIN

The skin is tough, stretchable and its thickness and structure differ in different parts of the body. It is thickest where it is most exposed, such as over the footpad and nose. It is also thicker over the back area (dorsal surface) and sides (lateral surface) of the body. The skin is thinnest over the ear flap, thorax, abdomen (ventral surface) and inner surface of the legs. Compared with human skin, the skin of the dog or cat is rather fragile. Without the protective cover of hair, its total thickness may be less than 1 mm in places on the body. The skin is composed of three layers (Fig. 5.1) and these are described below.

Epidermis

This is the non-vascular (i.e. lacks blood vessels) cellular layer composed of stratified epithelium. It is of varying thickness and forms the outer covering of the body. The epidermis consists of four layers of cells, from the basal layer, which is the deepest, to the top keratinised layer (Fig. 5.2).

In the basal layer (stratum basale or germinativum), the cells divide rapidly. The melanocytes are found between the cells of this layer. These cells are responsible for colour, as they contain the skin pigment melanin (in varying amounts). Heredity is the main factor that influences the colour of skin but, as with humans, sunlight and some hormones can also affect the skin colour. If melanin is not present the condition is called albinism and the animal may be called albino.

The next layer, known as the spinous layer (stratum spinosum), is one to two cells thick. It is thicker in body regions which undergo hard wear, such as

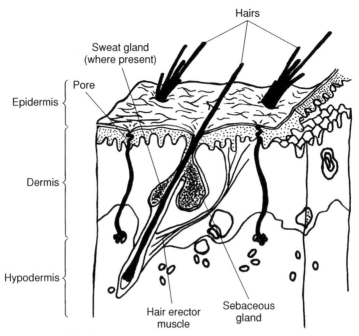

Fig. 5.1 Composition of the skin.

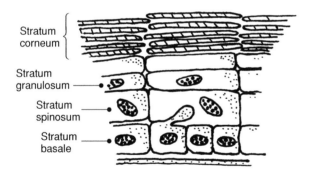

Fig. 5.2 The epidermal layers.

footpads in dogs. Next is the granular layer (stratum granulosum), so called because the cells have granules in the cytoplasm. It is in this layer that cells begin to die as they gradually move to the surface. Keratinisation begins in this layer as keratin, a fibrous protein, hardens the texture of the cells. In areas of hard wear on the body a clear layer is also found here. This layer gets its name from the loss of the cell nuclei and the tightly packed cells.

The top layer (stratum corneum) is made up of flat, cornified cells (dry scales), overlapping each other. If the scales remain intact, this top layer of cells prevents the entry of harmful materials. Keratinisation is completed here and gives the special epidermal parts of animals (hooves, beaks and hair) their strength. Dead cells from this layer are continuously sloughed off as dandruff or scurf, and replaced by new cells that come up from the basal layer.

Dermis (corium)

The dermis is made up of dense, fibrous, elastic, connective tissue, which contains blood vessels and nerves. The dermis also has bundles of involuntary muscle, called the arrector pili. These are attached to hair follicles, and when they contract, the hairs become more erect. The effect of this action is to increase the animal's insulation in cold weather. This involuntary muscle contraction has another function, seen in the sympathetic nervous system reaction 'fight or flight' – when the animal raises its 'hackles' (the hairs along the back and neck) it presents a larger and more frightening shape to an opponent.

Also found in the dermis are the sebaceous glands, sweat glands, and nerves which send information about sensation of touch, heat, cold and pain.

Hypodermis (subcutis)

The hypodermis contains connective tissue and fatty (adipose) tissue, allowing the skin to move over deeper structures without tearing or damage.

FUNCTIONS OF SKIN

Protection

- The skin acts as a barrier between the internal body environment and the external environment.
- It prevents entry of micro-organisms.
- It protects underlying structures from injury due to loss of water, mechanical trauma and ultraviolet light.
- It protects against absorption of toxic or harmful substances.

Production

- The skin produces vitamin D, which is required for the absorption of calcium from the intestines.
- Sebum is produced in the sebaceous glands and forms a water repellent layer over the skin, and also helps to control bacterial growth.
- The skin produces sweat, which assists in the removal of some waste products.
- Pheromones are produced from special scent glands, and are meant for communication with other animals for reproductive or territorial purposes.
- Milk is produced in the mammary glands.

Sensory

The skin is a sense organ with nerve receptors for touch, temperature, pressure and pain scattered throughout its surface.

Storage

The skin stores fat as adipose tissue. This is the body's energy store and serves as an insulation layer to help maintain body temperature in cold weather.

Temperature control (thermo-regulation)

- For losing heat the walls of the surface blood vessels widen (vasodilation) and sweat formed in the skin glands assists in the loss of water and salts by evaporating and cooling the skin surface.
- For gaining heat the walls of the surface blood vessels constrict or narrow (vasoconstriction), and erection of hairs traps a layer of air warmed by the skin for insulation.
- The fat layer (adipose tissue) under the skin also helps in the insulation of the body. It is situated in the subcutaneous layer called the hypodermis (see above).

Communication

- Pheromones. These are scents produced by special skin glands and used for communication with other animals, such as to attract another animal for reproductive purposes.
- Visual communication or camouflage involves the coat colour or pattern.
- In response to a threat or an attack, the coat hairs will become erect (raising its 'hackles') so that the animal appears to be larger. These hackles are seen especially in the neck and spine area.

SKIN GLANDS

Glands in the skin produce a variety of secretions:

- **Sebaceous glands** surround the hair follicles and secrete sebum, whose function is to form a thin, oily, water-repellent layer over the skin surface (Fig. 5.3). It gives the coat hair a shiny glossy appearance and helps to prevent bacterial growth on the skin's surface, which might in turn lead to infection. Some non-castrated cats may develop a greasy matting of the fur at the base of the tail due to overactive sebaceous glands, called a stud tail. This over-secretion of the tail glands is normal in some male dogs and is seen as greasy deposits on the skin's surface, often with a distinctive rancid smell. Wire-haired breeds of dog are particularly susceptible to this, e.g. West Highland White Terrier.
- **Apocrine sweat glands** open either into the hair follicle or onto the skin's surface. Their secretions do not help with control of body temperature nor do they allow moisture loss. These secretions contain some waste from the body, hence their smell is used by cats in particular to mark their territory. In dogs these glands are concentrated in regions such as the anal sacs. A particular dog/cat

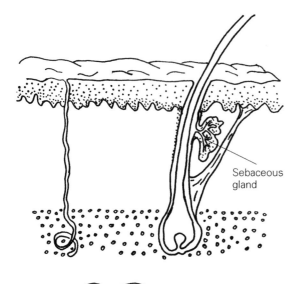

Fig. 5.3 Sebaceous gland in the skin.

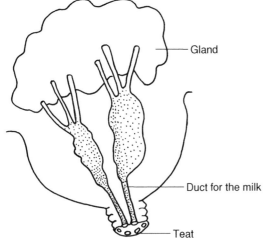

Gland

Duct for the milk

Teat

Fig. 5.4 Mammary gland.

odour is produced when the secretions are broken down by bacteria in the skin's surface.

- **Eccrine sweat glands**, useful for body cooling, are found only on the footpads and nose of both dog and cat.
- **Anal glands** or anal sacs are found on either side of the anus, positioned at 4 o'clock and 8 o'clock. Their secretion has an unpleasant smell and is thought to be a pheromone for marking territory. These sacs are intermittently emptied by the animal when passing faeces (see Fig. 3.11, Chapter 3).
- **Mammary glands** are modified skin glands and their function is to produce milk (Fig. 5.4). They are a feature of mammals and are found on the surface of the abdomen. Normally, the dog has five paired glands and the cat has four paired glands. The glands are present in both male and female animals but only enlarge with milk at the end of pregnancy.

NAILS, CLAWS AND FOOTPADS

Nails and claws

Nails and claws are modified or specialised epidermis (outer layer of skin), covered by a fold of skin. They are beak-like in shape, growing in two sheets which form the walls of the claw. In the middle of the nail or claw is the dermis, which contains a blood vessel and nerve between the last bone of the toe and the horn of the nail/claw. The sole, the part that the faces the ground when the animal is standing, is a soft flaky horn, with the wall of the nail/claw sometimes meeting and covering it (Fig. 5.5). The functions of nails and claws include:

- Bearing the weight of the animal and so assisting in movement.
- Obtaining food.
- Fighting, especially in cats.

Each of the four toes or digits of the animal's foot has a nail or claw, and some dogs may have a fifth toe on the inside surface of the lower leg known as the dew nail. The cat has a fifth toe on its front feet only. Claws usually wear down by weight bearing on hard surfaces (e.g. walking on pavements). Cats' claws are narrower than dog nails and are usually kept pulled back, off the ground, in the skin fold by ligaments. The claws can be quickly unsheathed by muscular action when required. Fig. 5.6 shows a typical dog and cat foot.

Footpads

A footpad forms the weight-bearing surface of the animal's foot. The footpad consists of specialised hairless skin, which is thick and normally pigmented and

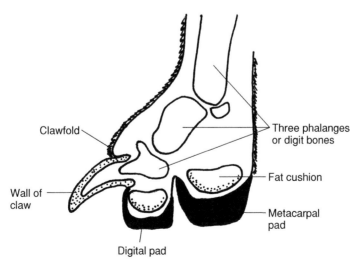

Fig. 5.5 Lateral view of a foot showing claw, pad and bone.

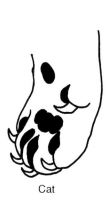
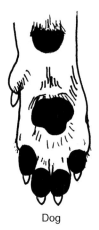

Cat   Dog

Fig. 5.6 Typical forefoot showing claw and pad of the dog and cat.

sweat glands are present. Under this is the toe or digital cushion made up of fatty or adipose tissue and a good blood supply. The pad is oval or heart shaped, depending on location in the dog, and is more rounded in the cat. The cat also has a single carpal pad which lies above the other pads on the foot. The pads give support to the feet and act as shock absorbers when running on all sorts of surfaces and landing from a leap or jump.

COAT GROWTH

Hair is an epidermal structure and its growth is controlled by:

- Seasons
- Environment
- Nutrition
- Hormones

In carnivores, the rhythm of shedding occurs independently in each hair follicle. The coat is thickest in winter, and normally some shedding occurs in spring and summer (animals living in a house may shed hair all year due to the central heating simulating summer). The pattern varies from breed to breed. In some breeds, such as the poodle, the hair grows continuously and needs regular clipping whereas in short haired breeds of dog new hairs grow and old ones are shed.

Hair growth is slow in summer, the rate increasing as the temperatures gets cooler in autumn and winter. During active growth, about 1 mm of hair shaft grows per week but this can be affected by hormonal changes. Once a hair stops growing it dies while it is still in the follicle. After that it can be shed from the skin at any time, and another hair is produced from the deep epidermal cells.

Dog and cat coats consist of 'guard' hairs with clusters of two to five compound follicles, each containing approximately three coarse primary hairs, which are larger and stiffer, with 6–12 secondary hairs, which are smaller and softer and are called under-hairs. There are common openings on the surface of the skin for the groups of hairs. The compound follicles cover most of the skin surface, and the arrangement and pattern varies from breed to breed. The number of hairs in a group varies with the type of hair coat. For example, in the Labrador retriever each group consists of a central primary guard hair and a number of thinner secondary hairs which form the undercoat, but in the Boxer, the coat consists of many small primary hairs and little undercoat. Generally, on the dorsal and lateral sides of the dog and cat there are many hairs, giving a thick coat; however, the coat on the abdomen is much thinner, as also under the tail and the inner surface of the flank. In some breeds there are no hairs or only a few in the anal region or on the testicles.

Formation of a hair

The hair growth cycle has three phases:

(1) Anagen: This is the most active stage of hair growth. The epidermis thickens (Fig. 5.7) and starts to grow into the dermis below (Fig. 5.8). This is the hair papilla. Epithelial cells produce a hair cone which later forms the actual hair (Fig. 5.9). Once a hair has reached its optimum length, it stops growing (Fig. 5.10).
(2) Catagen: The fully grown hair is still attached to the papilla (Fig. 5.10).
(3) Telogen: The papilla contracts, loosening the hair (Fig. 5.11) and begins to grow a new one (Fig. 5.12). The old hair is frequently pushed out by the new growth.

The three phases occur in different parts of the body at different times of year. Coat hair moults in spring and autumn and this lasts for about six weeks. The new coat hair is fully in place after four months.

Not all breeds of dog and cat follow this cycle. These breeds are called non-shedding breeds, e.g. Poodle and Rex cat.

Functions of coat hair are:

• Protection from injury
• Insulation in cold weather
• Colour/identification of a breed
• Sensory

Specialised or sensory hair is also called tactile hair, e.g. lower and upper eyelashes (superciliary and cilia), external ear hair (tragic or tragus), and whiskers on the muzzle (vibrissae). These hairs are more than twice as thick as guard hairs (Fig. 5.13). All the special hairs have deeper follicles with greater blood and nerve supply. When the animal moves between objects the hairs act as sensory organs

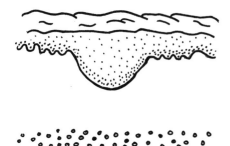

Fig. 5.7   The thickening epidermis.

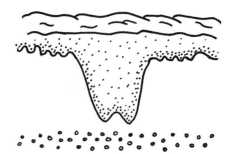

Fig. 5.8   Epidermal extension growing into a section of the dermis to form the hair papilla.

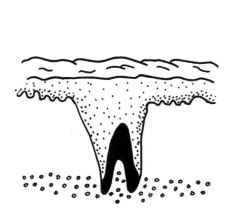

Fig. 5.9   Anagen.

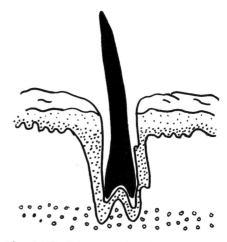

Fig. 5.10   Late anagen to catagen.

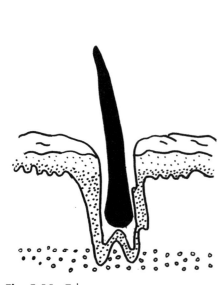

Fig. 5.11   Telogen.

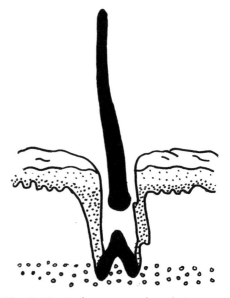

Fig. 5.12   Early anagen and new hair developing.

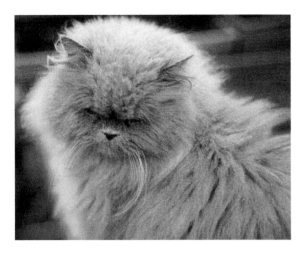

Fig. 5.13 Vibrissae and tragus hairs on a Persian cat.

and pick up information (pressure or touch) to indicate the position of the head and therefore of the body in relation to a given space for safe passage of the animal.

Both the coat and skin can be affected by disease, age, nutrition and parasites. Compared with other body organs, the skin is able to show a variety of signs and symptoms of ill health. These skin changes in themselves are not always of assistance in diagnosing the underlying disease because some diseases have similar symptoms. However, a change in the coat and skin condition is significant and should be reported so that veterinary investigations can be carried out.

Parasites, both internal and external, contribute to ill health in the animal host. Serious illness is rare but in cases of worm burden the host animal may appear unthrifty, i.e. the animal shows poor growth and anaemia.

PARASITOLOGY

A parasite lives in/on another living body and benefits by obtaining its nourishment from the host. The host can be any species, e.g. human, dog, cat, mouse or bird.

Terminology

- Transport host: This transports the parasite to the next host. No development takes place in the parasite.
- Paratenic host: It is same as transport, but the parasite must be eaten by this host in order to be excreted and passed on to the next host.
- Intermediate host: Some parasites must spend time in this host in order to enter their next life cycle stage.
- Final host: In this host the parasite completes its development.

- Permanent parasite: This parasite goes through all life stages and lives on one host.
- Temporary parasites: These move from host to host.
- Endoparasites: These live inside the host's body.
- Ectoparasites: These live on the surface of the host's body.

The parasite feeds on the host, but does not deliberately kill its host as this would destroy its food source. However, some hosts may die as a result of the parasite's feeding activities or from toxins released by the parasite. To prevent disease or death of the host animal, control of parasites is important. Control in dogs and cats aims to remove completely all parasites, whether internal or external.

Many easy to use and effective products are available for removing external parasites such as fleas, lice and ticks. These use a residue effect which lasts for varying periods of time. The products for eliminating internal parasites are collectively called wormers (anthelmintics).

Life cycles of common external parasites

The flea (Ctenocephalides; *Fig. 5.14)*

Fleas live mainly around the neck, ears, tail and abdomen and can cause the host animal to scratch and self-mutilate in an attempt to reduce the itching. Fleas feed exclusively on the blood they draw from the host animal. Flea faeces can be seen on the skin of affected animals as black hard dirt. If some of the black dirt grains are placed on a wet tissue the dried blood soon stains the tissue red. Many animals are allergic to flea saliva and this is manifested as irritation, scratching a specific area, inflammation and hair loss. Fleas are not host specific and will feed on any available host, including humans! Fleas are the intermediate host for the tapeworm, *Dipylidium caninum*, therefore worming may also be applicable when treating the host for a flea problem.

Life cycle

- Flea eggs hatch in 1–2 days.
- Flea larvae feed for 4–8 days (in carpets or bedding).

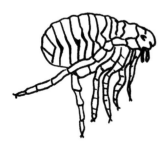

Fig. 5.14 Flea.

- The larvae spin cocoons, and adults emerge in five days or less.
- The adult flea cycle may take only three weeks; however, if the environment is not friendly (no host animal available) the larvae can remain unchanged for months before further development. Adult fleas can live for two years without feeding if food is unavailable.

The tick (Ixodes)

The tick will drop onto or climb into a host animal's coat and bury their mouth parts into the skin. They feed until engorged on the host blood before dropping on the ground. When engorged they appear grey to brown and are approximately pea sized. The adult tick (Fig 5.15) can live for two years without feeding.

Life cycle

- The engorged female can lay 1000–3000 eggs
- Larvae hatch in 30 days
- Nymphs emerge from moulted larvae
- Adult ticks emerge after 12 days, and immediately start to look for a blood meal

Feeding is required between each stage of development. When attempting to remove a tick, care must be taken not to pull the body leaving the mouth parts attached.

Diseases are transmitted by the tick to other host animals through its saliva and include:

- Lyme disease: This is a bacterial tick-borne infection caused by *Borrelia burg-dorferi*. The bacteria can cause skin discoloration, cardiac and joint disease in the infected animal. It is endemic in a number of states in the USA. In Europe, the bacteria are also borne by ticks of host wildlife such as rodents and deer. Signs of Lyme disease include:
  (a) sudden onset of lameness with arthritic pain in one or more joints (i.e. carpal or wrist joint), which may last only a few days and recur at intervals
  (b) high temperature with enlarged surface lymph nodes.

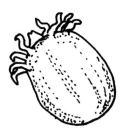

Fig. 5.15 Tick.

- Ehrlichiosis: This is caused by a parasite which lives inside certain white blood cells. It is transmitted by ticks during feeding on the host animal's blood. It is found in the Mediterranean basin in Europe and other Mediterranean countries. The severity of the disease and recovery of the host animal depends on the ability of its immune system. Certain breeds of dog are particularly susceptible to the disease, e.g. German shepherds. Babesiosis may also be present, having been passed by the tick at the same time. Signs of ehrlichiosis include:
  (a) high temperature and inappetence
  (b) enlarged lymph nodes
  (c) bleeding from the nose and under the skin
  (d) anaemia.
- Babesiosis: This is caused by a protozoon which develops and multiplies in tick salivary glands and it is transmitted to the host animal during feeding. It is endemic across much of Europe. The parasite protozoa infect red blood cells. The severity of the disease varies depending on the species and strain of *Babesia* and the health status of the animal infected. Signs of babesiosis include:
  (a) pale mucous membranes
  (b) anaemia
  (c) breathing problems and collapse.

Lice

There are two types of louse:

- Biting lice are visible to the eye and can be seen walking around on the skin when the coat hair is parted (5.16). They feed mainly on hair and dead skin (epithelial) cells of the host animal. *Trichodectes canis*, which infests dogs, is also one of the intermediate hosts for the internal parasitic worm *Dipylidium caninum*. The species infesting cats is called *Felicola subrostratus*.
- The sucking louse, *Linognathus*, infests dogs and feeds off the blood of the host animal (Fig. 5.17).

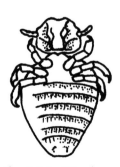

Fig. 5.16 Biting louse.

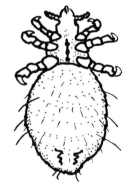

Fig. 5.17 Sucking louse.

Lice are permanent parasites, spending their entire life cycle on the host. During their lifespan of about a month, the adult female will lay up to 300 eggs. The eggs are known as nits and they stick (are cemented) to the hair shaft of the host's coat hair.

Life cycle

- Eggs are laid and are cemented to the coat hair.
- Three stages of nymph emerge (seen as smaller versions of the adult louse).
- Adults emerge three weeks after the last nymph moult.

Lice cause intense irritation and inflammation, and the host animal often self-inflicts skin injury during scratching. Severe infestations of lice may result in ill health and anaemia in young or weak animals, particularly if the blood-sucking louse *Linognathus setosus* is present.

Mites

Sarcoptes (Fig. 5.18)
The fertilised female burrows into the epidermis of the skin feeding on fluid from the damaged tissue, causing pain to the host animal. Sarcoptic mange is seen as intense inflammation and self-inflicted injury to the area, and results from scratching by the host animal. Crusts form in the bite area and hair is lost.

The areas most frequently affected initially are the edges of the ears, muzzle, face and elbows but later the rest of the body may become involved. *Sarcoptes* will infest humans and is manifested as itchy mosquito-like bites especially around the waist.

The sarcoptic mite may live for only 3–4 weeks in total. Its life cycle is as follows:

- Eggs are laid in tunnels within the epidermis of the skin.
- Larvae hatch in 3–5 days, crawling onto the skin surface to burrow into just the surface layers of skin forming 'moulting pockets'.

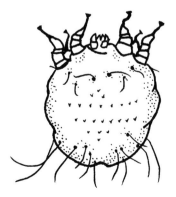

Fig. 5.18 *Sarcoptes.*

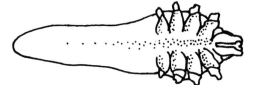

Fig. 5.19 *Demodex.*

- Nymphs follow through two nymph stages.
- Adult mites emerge, the full cycle taking about 17 days.

Demodex canis (Fig. 5.19)

Demodex is a long, cigar-shaped mite with short, stubby legs, living in the hair follicles and sebaceous skin glands of most mammals. Transmission between animals occurs only within the first few days of life between mother and young during suckling. The whole life cycle of *Demodex* is spent in the hair follicles or glands. It is also known as sub-surface follicular mite.

Demodex is seen in animals which become stressed or debilitated for any reason. Early signs of infection are some hair loss (alopecia) on the face, particularly around the eyes, and the forelegs. The skin often becomes noticeably thickened. There are two forms of infection:

- Mild, seen as skin inflammation, thickening and hair loss.
- Severe, with moist and dried discharge of serum and pus, a lot of inflammation and hair loss.

Cheyletiella (Fur mite; Fig. 5.20)

Cheyletiella, visible to the eye, is a permanent parasite, spending its entire life cycle on the host animal. It is host specific, but can affect humans. The mites live mainly on the surface of the skin and feed off epithelial skin cells, tissue and cellular fluid from the host. The host animal often has an allergic reaction to the mite saliva. Its life cycle is as follows:

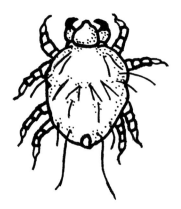

Fig. 5.20 *Cheyletiella.*

- Eggs are laid and cemented to coat hair similar to lice.
- Eggs hatch into six-legged larvae.
- These moult into eight-legged larvae.
- Adult stage is reached.

Cheyletiella cause skin irritation seen as excessive scurf or dandruff in the coat of the infected host animal. It is often referred to as walking dandruff and can affect both dog (*Cheyletiella yasguri*) and cat (*Cheyletiella blakei*).

Otodectes cynotis (Fig. 5.21)

Otodectes is also known as ear mite. It is not host specific and will infest cats, dogs and other small animals. The mites are found mostly in the external ear canal but may also occur around the tail and feet areas. They feed off the protective layer of wax in the host animal's ear canal, often damaging the canal lining. *Otodectes* is a permanent parasite spending its entire life cycle on the host with a life cycle of approximately three weeks:

- Eggs are laid.
- Larvae form.
- Two stages of nymph.
- Moulting to adults.

Otodectes mites cause head shaking and ear scratching. On examination of the ear canal a brownish, waxy secretion is seen in the ear canal. Often inflammation and bacterial infection is seen due to the damage caused to the lining of the canal by the feeding mites.

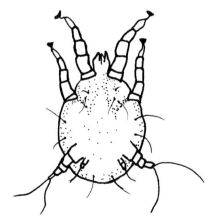

Fig. 5.21 *Otodectes.*

Trombicula autumnalis (Harvest mite; Fig. 5.22)

Harvest mites normally become a problem for a host animal in late summer and early autumn. The larval form of the mite attaches to the legs of a passing dog or

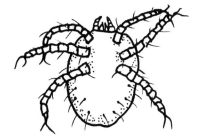

Fig. 5.22 Harvest mite larva.

cat. It is this form that is parasitic to both animals and humans and therefore not host specific. The mite is transmitted by direct contact of the host animal with foliage in fields or heavy undergrowth where the larvae crawl on hatching. They are bright orange and round in shape before feeding and have three pairs of legs. They localise on the ears, muzzle, feet and legs of the host to feed. The larvae bite the skin surface and inject an enzyme which will start to digest the host tissue enabling feeding by the mite. This causes inflammation and irritation for the host and is seen as self-trauma to the area as a result of scratching. The larvae feed for up to 15 days before dropping off to enter the nymph stage before the adult form.

Life cycles of common endoparasites

Endoparasites live inside the host animal. Most dogs and cats will have had worms of some sort during their lives. Routine treatment with wormers (anthelmintics) through the year by the owner will ensure that there is little sign of worms or inconvenience caused to the host animal. Host animals become infected by swallowing an egg or larval form of the endoparasite. The common endoparasites can be divided into two groups.

Roundworm (ascarids)

Roundworms have an un-segmented body with one alimentary tract (Fig. 5.23). The adults are yellow/white in colour and both ends are pointed. The adults live in the intestines of the host, feeding on digesting food in the gut. Female worms produce thousands of eggs which are passed during defaecation. These eggs are sticky therefore will attach to the feet and coat of animals, often being swallowed during grooming. The roundworms that infest dogs are *Toxocara canis* and *Toxascaris leonina*, and those that infest cats are *Toxocara cati* and *Toxascaris leonina*.

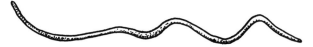

Fig. 5.23 Roundworm.

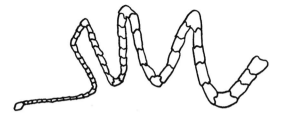

Fig. 5.24 Tapeworm.

Toxocara canis is transmissible to humans (zoonotic agent) and can migrate in human tissues. It is linked to blindness and the disease in humans is called toxocariasis.

Tapeworm (cestode)

Tapeworms have a flat, segmented body and each segment is independent, with its own alimentary tract (Fig. 5.24). They attach by the mouth to the intestinal wall of the host animal. Worm segments break off and are passed out with faeces, often attaching to the hair around the tail region of the host. They look like mobile grains of rice and cause considerable anal irritation. Fleas are the usual intermediate host for the worm eggs in the life cycle of the tapeworm. *Dipylidium caninum* infest dogs and cats and *Echinococcus granulosa* infestation is linked to dogs fed on raw meat. This tapeworm infests humans as a zoonotic agent and causes the disease hydatidosis or hydatid disease.

Other worm types in the dog and cat include whipworm (*Trichuris vulpis*) and hookworm (*Uncinaria stenocephala*).

An animal with worms will not always show signs of infestation. The following signs appear only if the infestation overwhelms the resistance of the host animal:

- Anal irritation, seen as scooting on bottom
- Constantly hungry, eating but losing weight
- Vomiting and diarrhoea
- Unhealthy, dull coat
- Enlarged abdomen (seen particularly in young animals)

Prevention of worms

- Worm animals regularly
- Control the intermediate hosts (flea and lice)
- Dispose of faeces immediately
- Disinfect where faeces have been
- Always wash hands thoroughly
- Wash animal bowls separately from human utensils
- Do not let animal lick face
- Keep animal's anal area clean
- Examine faeces regularly for signs of worm infestation

Other internal parasites

Protozoa

These are single-celled animals and range in size from microscopic to just visible to the naked eye. Prozotoa form a cyst at some point in their life cycle that enables them to pass from host to host and to survive temporarily outside a host animal. The diseases caused by protozoa include:

- Toxoplasmosis: This is caused by *Toxoplasma gondii*. Dogs (and sheep) normally become infected by eating contaminated cat faeces. Toxoplasma is linked to cats as the carrier. The cyst form is passed in their faeces which can then affect any species. It causes a zoonotic disease in humans and is particularly harmful to the unborn child during pregnancy.
- Coccidiosis: This is caused by *Coccidia* and results in diarrhoea in dogs who become infected after drinking contaminated water or when housed in crowded conditions.
- Leishmaniasis: This is caused by a protozoon which is transmitted by the Sand fly. It is endemic in the Mediterranean basin, the Middle East and many sub-tropical and tropical regions of the world. The parasite invades the white blood cells first then other body tissues. It is a zoonotic agent and the parasite has an incubation period which may be extremely long. Clinical features include weight loss, skin disease, joint pain, intermittent fever and kidney damage.

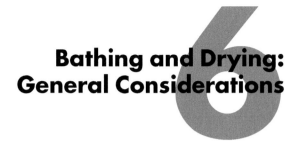

Bathing and Drying: General Considerations

DOGS

Your choice of bath depends on whether you are grooming commercially or just trimming your own dog at home. For salon purposes, baths specifically made for the professional groomer (Fig. 6.1) are available, some of which recycle the water. Alternatively, a human bath or a catering sink can be used. Whatever bath you choose, ensure that the height is set correctly for you to bath large or small dogs.

For grooming at home, obviously the choice is yours whether you wish to bath the dog in your own bath or sink, or if you wish to buy one specifically for the purpose. However, remember to ensure that the bath has a non-slip bottom for the dog's protection.

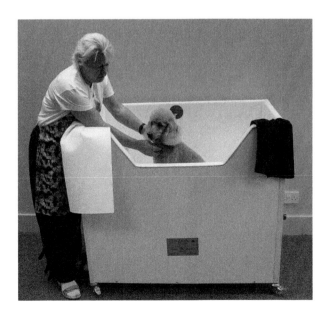

Fig. 6.1 A groomer's purpose-built bath that uses recycled water.

Before you start bathing your dog it is essential that all the equipment is at hand so that you do not leave the dog unattended. The equipment required includes shampoo, conditioner, sponge, bucket, moisture absorbent cloth, towels and bathing restraints. (Figs 6.2 and 6.3)

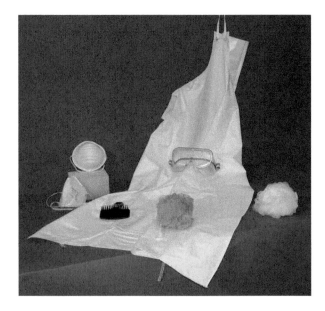

Fig. 6.2 Protective clothing and shampoo applicators.

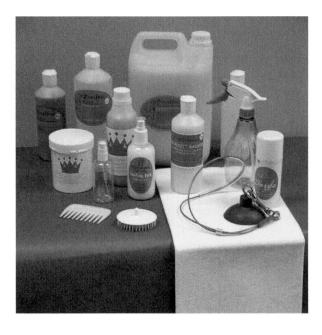

Fig. 6.3 Shampoos, absorbent cloth and restrainer.

Shampoos and conditioners

There are five main types of shampoo:

- Cleansing: These contain a strong substance that acts against grease and dirt.
- Mild: These remove grease and dirt, leaving in some of the natural oils.
- Medicated: These contain mild anti-bacterial products that act on the skin.
- Veterinary: These are prescribed by vets for particular skin conditions.
- Insecticidal: These kill parasites.

Although many different types of shampoo are available for all the different coat types and colours, they will all fit into one of the above mentioned categories. A shampoo should be used according to the manufacturer's instructions, but it is generally diluted. Occasionally you may have dogs that are very greasy or particularly dirty and here a tiny amount of washing-up liquid or undiluted shampoo can be helpful. Use washing-up liquid *only* as a last resort as the coat will be stripped of its natural oils.

Again several makes of conditioner are available. Trial and usage or recommendation is the only way to discover what suits a dog's coat. Do not over-use conditioner and ensure it is rinsed out thoroughly, otherwise the coat will be left greasy.

Bathing procedure

Most dogs are happy to be bathed as long as it is done with care. There are some that react badly to the shower so do not keep the pressure too high. Bathing can be done as often as you like provided a good-quality shampoo is used to replenish the natural oils. As mentioned previously, bathing of wire coats is not recommended; other methods of cleaning the coat are discussed in Chapter 11 (Breed profiles). When bathing a dog always work to a routine to ensure that the job is done thoroughly.

- Check the water temperature on the inside of your wrist to make sure it is at the body temperature.
- Prepare the shampoo.
- Place the dog in the bath (ensure safety by using a rubber mat in the bottom of the bath and a bath fastener).
- Wet the dog thoroughly, keeping the shower head close to the body, starting behind the shoulders and working back over the body, down the legs and tail and then finally the head. This method will help with dogs that are nervous because you are not alarming them by going straight around the eyes and ears. Work the water through the coat to ensure total saturation; this is particularly important for heavy, thick coats. Take care not to let the water go into the ears or nose. It is possible for a small dog or short-nosed dog to drown by water entering the nasal passages and going into the lungs. Water in the ear canal can cause irritation.
- Check and empty the anal glands if necessary (see Chapter 3).

- Apply shampoo using a sponge as this creates a better lather – the lather shows that the shampoo is working. Begin shampooing at the tail to remove any residue from the glands. Shampoo down each back leg to the foot (Fig. 6.4).

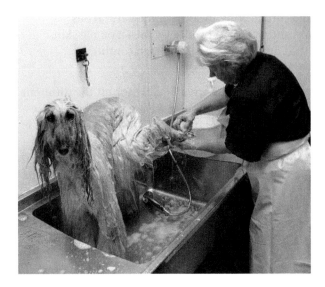

Fig. 6.4 Applying shampoo to the back leg.

- Shampoo the body and undercarriage, the front legs, feet, shoulders and chest and then finally apply the shampoo carefully to the head (Fig. 6.5). Cover the eyes to ensure that no shampoo goes in and wipe any excess suds away with your thumb. Remember to thoroughly wash the beard. By shampooing the head last there is less of a chance of shampoo going in the eyes; it may also stop the dog from shaking itself.

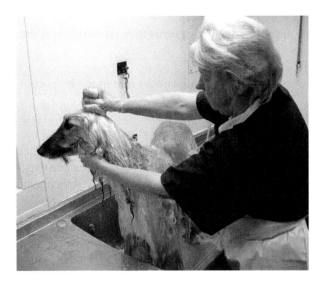

Fig. 6.5 Applying shampoo carefully to head.

- Rinse the dog from head to tail using your hand to push the suds and water through the coat (Fig. 6.6). It is usually necessary to shampoo a dog twice to ensure that the coat is thoroughly cleaned so the first rinse can be done quickly.

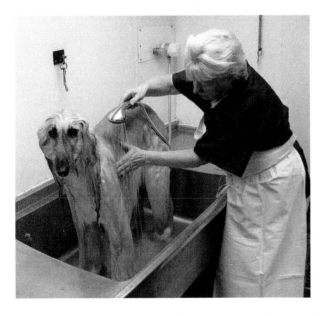

Fig. 6.6 Push the water through the coat.

- Apply shampoo again in the same way as described above.
- Rinse thoroughly, ensuring that the coat 'squeaks' as you push the water through (see Fig. 6.6). The squeaking sound means that all the suds are removed and this is vitally important as a residue can result in a dull, lifeless coat and possibly skin irritation.
- Apply conditioner to the coat if appropriate (see Chapter 9 for shampooing and conditioning for different coat types).
- Rinse thoroughly.
- Squeeze the excess water from the coat with your hands or use a moisture absorbent cloth.
- Towel dry the dog.

Drying

There are various pieces of equipment for drying dogs depending on whether you are grooming your own pet or grooming commercially. Drying is done to:

- Dry the coat thoroughly
- Remove any knots or tangles
- Remove the dead undercoat

During drying, always keep your eyes open for lumps or bumps on the skin, any rashes or differences in coat texture. These basic signs could indicate an underlying problem – so here you can be an early warning system for the vet.

Equipment for drying

- Moisture absorbent cloths
- Towels
- High velocity dryer (blasters)
- Hand-held dryer
- Stand dryers
- Cage dryer
- Cabinet dryer

Towel drying

Towels or moisture absorbent cloths will remove excess water from the coat. The advantage of moisture absorbent cloths is that they can be wrung out and used again whereas towels hold the water. The usual commercial practice is to squeeze the excess water out of the coat with moisture absorbent cloth first and then towel dry. For most breeds further drying will be required; however, some smooth coats can be completely dried this way (see Chapter 9).

When using these items, ensure that you are firm with your actions but do not over-rub the coat as this may cause long coats to tangle. Once this stage is complete you should not be able to squeeze water from the coat.

Other methods of drying

High velocity dryers (blasters; Fig. 6.7)

This piece of equipment is a must in a busy commercial salon as the drying time can be reduced dramatically. The power from the machine 'blasts' the excess water and dead undercoat from the dog and separates the coat. However, some dogs may not like the sound or force of the blaster and if they object they should not be forced as this could genuinely frighten them. There are specific uses for different coat types that will be discussed in Chapter 9. Ideally, the groomer should wear goggles or face mask while using this equipment as loose hair and dead skin scales can cause eye irritation and inhalation of hair can lead to chest problems. However, this will only occur after very many uses!

The blaster should be used cautiously with a dog that has not met this equipment before. Introduce the machine at the lowest setting and always from the back end of the dog. Keep the nozzle close to the skin. If the dog is comfortable with this, gradually move up the body leaving the head until last. If the dog again is comfortable, increase the power setting but if it is not happy then go back to the low setting. Always use the blaster in an up-and-down or side-to-side motion and never in circles. If the blaster is used in the correct way it will divide and separate the coat and not tangle it (Fig. 6.8). Continue working the coat until it is separated and water does not blow from it (Fig. 6.9). If the dog is accepting the blaster all over the body, you can try to blast very carefully around the head; cover the dog's

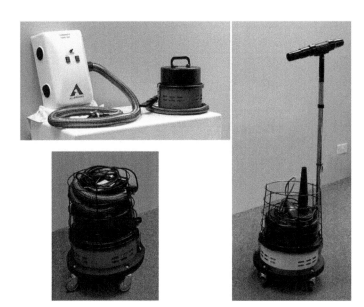

Fig. 6.7 High velocity dryers (blasters).

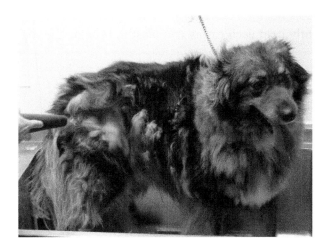

Fig. 6.8 Using a blaster.

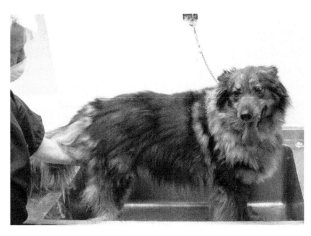

Fig. 6.9 Coat after blasting.

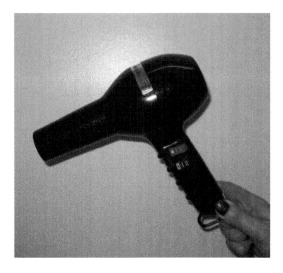

Fig. 6.10 Hand-held dryer.

eyes with your hands and gently hold each ear as you blast it, keeping the ear canal covered.

Hand-held dryers (Fig. 6.10)

These dryers are best known as 'human' dryers. They can be a useful extra dryer in a professional salon for drying small damp areas or difficult-to-reach areas on large dogs, e.g. armpits. If grooming at home, the hand-held dryer has the advantage for the pet owner of being economical to buy, but they are difficult to use as the dog cannot be brushed at the same time. Special holding arms can be purchased for this purpose, but this is definitely not the easiest or quickest way to dry your dog!

Stand dryers (Fig. 6.11)

These are most commonly used in the commercial salon and, as the name suggests, they comprise a dryer on a stand. Usually they have powerful motors with variable heat and speed settings, and their height is adjustable. The major advantage of these dryers is that your hands are free to use the brush at the same time as drying, which is vital for certain breeds such as Poodles (Ut-Wo) or Bichon Frise (To-Wo). Specific uses of stand dryers are covered in Chapter 9.

Cage and cabinet dryers (Fig. 6.12)

With these two drying methods the principle is the same – the dog is enclosed in a secure area with warm air circulating around it. A cage dryer is usually attached to a normal metal dog crate. A cabinet dryer is a specifically designed unit with a

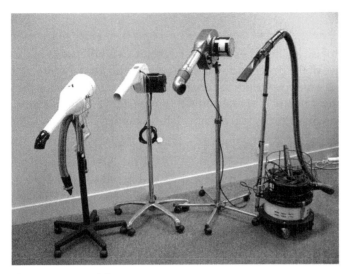

Fig. 6.11 Stand dryers.

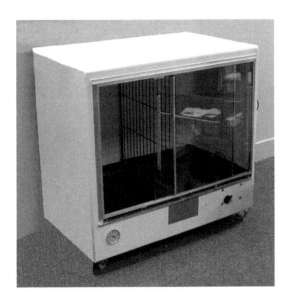

Fig. 6.12 Cabinet dryer.

fan circulating air and a temperature gauge to ensure the safety and comfort of the dog. Both methods should be monitored closely as a dog could get over-heated if left for too long at a time in the dryer. However, most elderly dogs and many cats enjoy the comfort of a sleep in the warm surroundings and quite often it is difficult to get them out! In a salon situation, the cabinet dryer is best used in conjunction with a high velocity dryer to minimise drying time.

CATS

Before bathing a cat, try to use a hair dryer on it first as some cats will not tolerate either the force or the noise of the dryer and you will end up with a soggy cat.

For bathing a cat, select an appropriate cat shampoo as not all shampoos are suitable for them due to the sensitivity of their skin. It is important to have all your equipment at hand before you begin as you cannot fasten a cat in the bath.

- Hold the cat by the scruff of the neck and if it wants to, let it rest its front feet on the edge of the bath.
- Rinse the coat, keeping the shower hose close to the skin, ensuring that the water is warm. It is important that the water is not cold as cats cannot tolerate cold water. *Do not* wet the cat's head because if water enters the ears of a cat it can cause serious problems.
- Start shampooing from the neck, down the body, to the tail. Pay particular attention to the base of the tail, as this area can be very greasy. Shampoo the legs, remembering to wash the feet (Fig. 6.13). Rinse thoroughly. Wipe around each ear and each eye using four separate pieces of damp cotton wool.

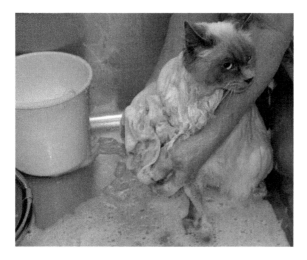

Fig. 6.13 Washing a cat's feet.

- Squeeze the excess water from the coat with a moisture absorbent cloth (Figs 6.14 and 6.15). Some cats will tolerate the blaster, which can be used after placing the cat in a basket or on a towel (Fig. 6.16). Then towel dry thoroughly (Fig. 6.17).

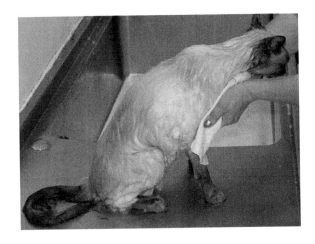

Fig. 6.14 Squeeze the excess water.

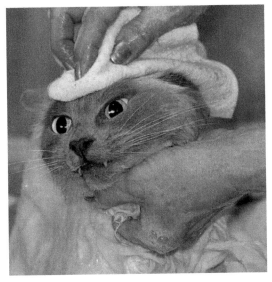

Fig. 6.15 Wiping the cat's head.

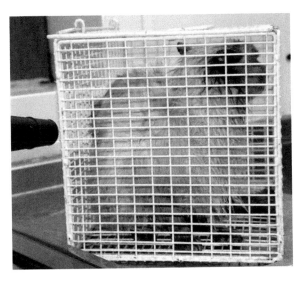

Fig. 6.16 Blasting the cat while it is sitting in a basket.

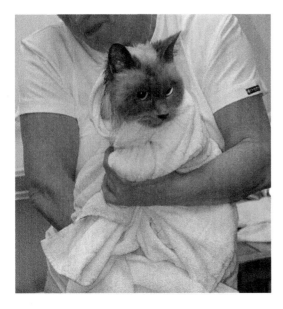

Fig. 6.17 Towel dry thoroughly.

• Cabinet drying is great for cats as they love the warmth but if you do not have a cabinet available, use a stand dryer and comb or brush the coat to remove all tangles and dead coat. A soft slicker brush (Fig. 6.18) could be used gently on the legs but remember that a cat's skin is much thinner and more sensitive than a dog's, so do not be harsh.

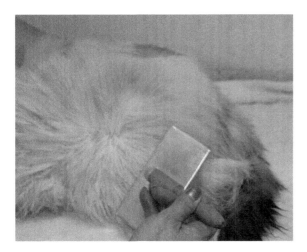

Fig. 6.18 Use a brush to brush the coat.

- If a cabinet is being used, remove the cat after ten minutes, comb through, and if the coat is still wet, return it to the cabinet for another ten minutes. Always finish with a stand dryer and comb to ensure thorough dryness and the complete removal of dead coat and knots.

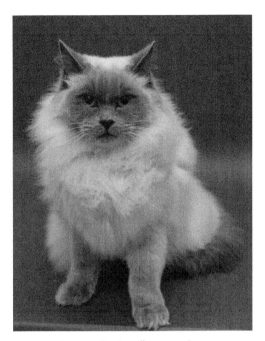

Fig. 6.19   A well-groomed cat.

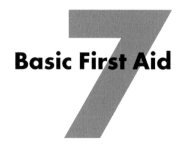

Basic First Aid

AIMS AND OBJECTIVES

First aid is the emergency care and treatment given to an animal which has suddenly fallen ill or suffered an injury, before medical/surgical care (veterinary treatment) can be commenced. The main objectives of first aid are to:

- Keep the animal alive
- Make it comfortable
- Assist in pain control
- Prevent it getting worse

Different situations require a different approach. It is essential to assess the situation quickly by asking yourself the following questions:

- Is the animal in further danger?
- Will you be in danger if you help?
- Can the animal be restrained?
- Can you move the animal from further risk or harm safely?

In some situations there is plenty of time to attend to the injuries or problems and the situations will not be life threatening. Other situations may be so severe that the animal will die if urgent and skilled emergency care is not available.

First aid, which involves only the initial actions of someone attending or witnessing an accident is very limited. It does not involve diagnosis or medical treatment of injuries, but is designed to preserve life; temporarily prevent a condition from getting worse if possible; and allow time to get the animal to the veterinary surgeon, who can then diagnose the full extent of the condition, which is not always obvious.

EVALUATION

VERY SEVERE – Must act immediately or the animal will die. Examples are:

- The heart has stopped (cardiopulmonary arrest).
- Breathing is obstructed due to an object in the air passages.

- Breathing has stopped.
- Bleeding from a main artery or vein.
- Acute allergic reaction to an insect sting or other substance.

SEVERE – Must act within one hour or the animal may die. Examples are:

- Deep cuts with considerable blood loss.
- Established shock.
- Head injuries.
- Breathing difficulties.

SERIOUS – Must act within 4–5 hours otherwise more serious problems will develop, which could be life threatening. Examples are:

- Bone fractures that puncture the skin (compound fractures).
- Spinal injuries.
- Early stages of shock.
- Difficulties in giving birth (dystocia).

MAJOR – Must act within 24 hours to prevent further damage. Examples are:

- Fractures with no skin injury (simple fractures)
- Prolonged vomiting and diarrhoea
- Foreign bodies in the eyes or ears

INITIAL MANAGEMENT

(1) **Assess the situation and keep calm**. Briefly examine the animal and note any obvious injuries.
(2) **Contact the veterinary practice** for advice and to let them know that you are coming.
(3) **Ensure your own safety**. Make sure the animal is properly restrained before handling and lifting, so that no one is bitten.
(4) **Stop and cover any obvious bleeding**. Use sterile dressings if possible to prevent further contamination.
(5) **Make sure the animal is able to breathe**. If the airway is obstructed try to clear it.
(6) **Treat for shock** by maintaining the body temperature.

HANDLING AND TRANSPORT

If the animal's life is in danger, then it must be moved. Injured animals are usually in pain, and they are shocked and frightened. This means they may attack any one who tries to approach or handle them. To protect both the handler and the animal from further harm or injury great care is needed at this time:

- Slow, deliberate movements are essential.
- A calm soothing voice will help in approaching the animal.
- Handle the animal as little as possible.
- Muzzle if necessary, but *only* if the animal has no breathing difficulties.

Transport the animal to the veterinary surgery, supporting any obvious injury, e.g. a fractured limb. However, before moving the animal, quickly assess the condition. This is referred to as 'initial help', and if it is done as soon as possible, the chances of survival are greatly improved. Checks that should be made during the initial help are listed below.

- Check airway – to ensure it is not obstructed; if it is check if can be cleared.
- Check breathing – to ensure that the animal can breathe and to assist with artificial respiration if required.
- Check heart and pulse – check the beat rate and strength and record these. If the heart has stopped then proceed with heart massage.

The initial assessment and help given must be reported to the veterinary staff on arrival at the surgery to reduce delays in the treatment of the injured animal.

Transport

Small dogs and cats

Transport small dogs and cats in a pet carrier or in a cat-sized basket making sure there are plenty of breathing holes. Many owners nowadays have a cat cage, which is ideal for small dogs, provided there is plenty of space to stretch out (Fig. 7.1). Otherwise the animal can be held in the owner's arms depending on the injury (Fig. 7.2).

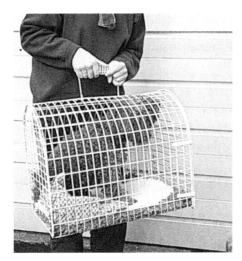

Fig. 7.1 Cat carrier for small dog or cat.

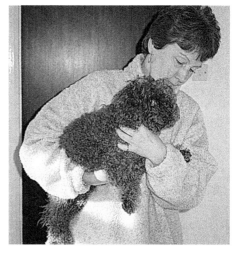

Fig. 7.2 Small injured dog being held in the arms.

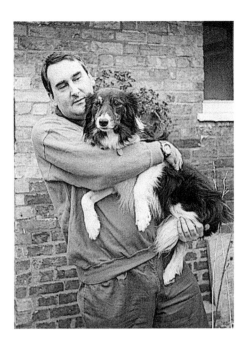

Fig. 7.3 Medium-sized dog held against the body for support.

Medium-sized dogs

If these dogs have only minor injuries they may be encouraged to walk slowly. If they not able to walk, put one arm around the front of the forelegs and the other arm around the hind legs (provided this is not contra-indicated by the injuries) and lift and hold close to the handler's body, with the legs free and hanging downwards (Fig. 7.3).

Large and giant breeds of dog

These animals should be lifted only by two or more people, one supporting the head and chest and another supporting the abdomen and hind quarters. If the animal is too large to be lifted up, with two or more handlers use a stretcher or blanket lift (Fig. 7.4). Pull the animal onto the blanket, laying it on its side, and lift up using the corners of the blanket. If there are not enough handlers available, simply drag the blanket, provided that the surface is smooth. The blanket lift can also be used for smaller dogs with spinal injuries (Fig. 7.5).

Safe lifting

Whatever the size of the injured animal it is important to always lift in the correct manner. Bend your knees before lifting, rather than bending from the waist. In this way, the handler's own back is less at risk, but if in doubt get more help (Fig. 7.6). As in human first aid, in animal first aid there is a **recovery position** in which the animal should be placed. Unless contra-indicated, this is the safe

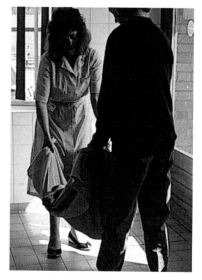

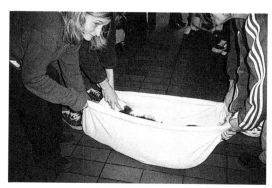

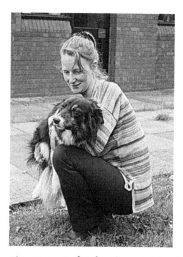

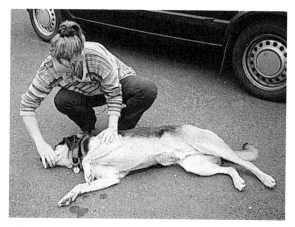

Fig. 7.4 (*Left*) Blanket lift requires two or more people.
Fig. 7.5 (*Right*) Animals with suspected spinal injuries can be transported in a blanket lift.

Fig. 7.6 (*Left*) Lift with straight back and bent knees to prevent handler's back injury.
Fig. 7.7 (*Right*) Recovery position for an injured animal, keeping the airway straight.

position in which the animal should be placed to ensure breathing is assisted and the heart is exposed for emergency procedures if required (Fig. 7.7). To put the animal in recovery position:

- Lay the animal on its right side.
- Straighten the head and neck.
- Pull the tongue forwards, behind the canine teeth or to one side of the mouth.
- Remove any collar or harness.

CHECKS AND OBSERVATIONS

- Any signs of bleeding from the animal's surface or from a body opening, e.g. the mouth, rectum, vulva, prepuce or ears.
- 'Colour check' by looking at the lining of the lower eyelid and the mucous membrane of the mouth and gums.

> **'Colour check' of mucous membranes**
> - **Pale**: Indicates shock or serious bleeding (internal or external)
> - **Blue**: Also referred to as cyanotic and indicates lack of oxygen to the tissue cells
> - **Yellow**: Also referred to as jaundice, can be caused by an excess of bile pigment in the bloodstream and usually involves the liver in some way
> - **Red/congested**: Indicates over-oxygenation after exercise, a heat stroke or a feverous condition

- The capillary refill time. The upper lip is lifted, and the gum over an upper canine tooth is pressed (Fig. 7.8). This squeezes the blood out of the surface capillaries, causing the area to go temporarily white. The refill time is the time it takes to become the normal pink colour again as the capillaries again fill up. Normal refill time is 1–1.5 seconds. Any time longer than this is considered as 'slow' and is reported; it may indicate a degree of shock.
- Rate and quality of the pulse. This is normally checked in the groin area of the hind leg on the femoral artery. Rate refers to the speed of the pulse which is a reflection of the heart beat. The pulse should be taken for a full minute for a true recording. The quality of the pulse refers to descriptions such as strong, thready, weak or normal. In order to describe this, the handler must have some experience of pulse taking.

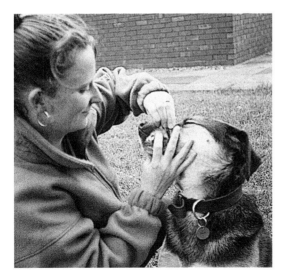

Fig. 7.8 Check capillary refill time by pressing the gum over an upper canine tooth.

- The rate of breathing is recorded and noted whether it is normal speed, slow, fast or shallow.
- Body temperature is checked by feeling the extremities of the body such as the feet and tail end. If the temperature is higher or lower than it should be the handler will be aware of the warmth or chill of the extremity being held.
- Record the animal's level of consciousness. In other words, can the animal respond to any stimuli like its name, a noise or sudden movement?
- Record any unusual odours from the animal's body and whether it is coming from the animal's mouth, anus or coat.

When assessing a sick or injured animal, the pulse recordings, a general idea of body temperature and the breathing rate will provide information about the:

- Body's ability to control body temperature.
- Heart's ability to pump the blood in the circulation to reach all body cells.
- Circulation's ability to transport the blood efficiently.
- Respiratory system's ability to supply the body oxygen requirement.

Temperature

A fall in temperature may be seen in:

- Shock and severe bleeding
- Impending death (moribund animal)
- Immediately before parturition

The temperature can be assessed with a thermometer, or by touching the extremities (feet), or by noting the body position (curled up or spread out). Normal body temperature as checked by thermometer is:

- Dog: 38.3–38.7°C (100.9–101.7°F)
- Cat: 38.0–38.5°C (100.4–101.6°F)

Pulse

Pulse is a means of checking the heart (cardio) and blood (vascular) function. With each heart beat, the walls of the arteries expand and contract in size to allow the created wave of blood to pass and to maintain its speed of flow – this is called the pulse. If there is a change in the heart function or in the volume of blood flowing in the blood vessels, there will be a corresponding change in the pulse rate (speed) or character. It is essential for the operator to spend some time practising feeling pulses, both normal and abnormal, to improve their skill. This will also dramatically decrease the time it takes the operator to find the animal's pulse. Descriptive words that are used to describe the pulse include:

- Intermittent
- Thready – slow, soft pulse

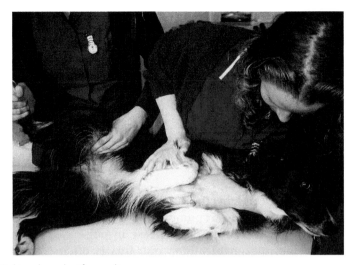

Fig. 7.9 Taking the pulse (femoral).

- Irregular
- Strong
- Weak

A normal pulse is described as regular, strong or firm. The pulse is taken where an artery runs close to the body surface. Each pulsation corresponds with the contraction of the right and left ventricles of the heart. The sites include the:

- Femoral artery located in the groin region on the medial aspect of the femur of the hind leg.
- Digital artery located on the cranial or anterior surface of the hock region of the hind leg.
- Coccygeal artery located on the ventral aspect (under-side) of the base of the tail just above the rectum.

The commonest site for taking the pulse is the femoral artery (Fig. 7.9) on the hind leg. Before taking the pulse the animal must be suitably restrained, therefore two people make the task much easier.

Taking the pulse

(1) Wait for the animal to get used to being restrained.
(2) Once the animal is settled, take the pulse by placing the fingers over the chosen artery.
(3) When properly located, using a watch with a 'second' hand, count the pulse for one minute. Never shorten this period because the pulse can change quickly and a reading of less than one minute could be inaccurate and therefore useless.

(4) Write down the pulse count at the end of the minute.
(5) Relax the restraint of the animal and praise it.

Normal pulse rates are:

• Dog*: 60–180 beats per minute
• Cat: 110–180 beats per minute

*The wide pulse range in dogs is due to the variation in size from toy breeds (nearer the upper (180) end of the range) to giant breeds (nearer the lower (60) end of the range).

Terms to describe the pulse are:

• **Dysrhythmia**: This indicates that the pulse and heart rate are not synchronised. The pulse is lower due to the heart pumping blood inefficiently.
• **Sinus arrhythmia**: This refers to the increase in pulse rate on breathing in and decrease in the rate on breathing out; this is often considered to be normal.
• **Fast pulse**: This occurs when the tissues are not getting enough oxygen and the heart is compensating by speeding up to meet the body's needs. A fast pulse is normal after exercise.

The pulse increases because of:

• Exercise
• Excitement or stress
• Heart/heart valve disease
• Shock or loss of blood
• Pain
• High temperature/fever

The pulse decreases because of:

• Sleep
• Unconsciousness
• Heart disease

Respiration

Normal breathing is almost silent, although air flow may be heard in the airways. The breathing, heart and circulatory system are very closely linked therefore a change in one is mirrored by a change in the other. If the blood gas levels of oxygen or carbon dioxide become abnormal this will be seen in the animal's colour, its pulse rate and character and in the breathing. Some breeds of dog and cat (short-nosed breeds), because of the anatomy of the airway, may make considerable breathing sounds; this is normal.

There should be a rhythm to the breathing, i.e. the time between breathing in and out should be equal. The breathing can be varied by use of the voluntary or skeletal muscles of the chest (thorax). It is because of the voluntary ability to alter breathing that the pulse should only be taken once the animal has settled. Any obvious restraint will probably cause the breathing to increase as a response.

The reading is taken either on breathing in or when the animal breathes out. It should *not* be taken when the animal:

- Is panting (cause for concern when seen in a cat)
- Has recently exercised
- Has been stressed by restraint
- Is asleep

Normal rates of breathing are:

- Dog: 10–30 breaths per minute
- Cat: 20–30 breaths per minute

It is timed using a watch with a second hand for one minute, also making note of the depth of the breathing.

Breathing may increase because of:

- Shock or bleeding
- Recent exercise
- Pain
- Excitement
- Heat stroke

Breathing may decrease because of:

- Unconsciousness
- Sleep
- Poisons
- Low body temperature (hypothermia)

Terms to describe breathing are:

- **Tachypnoea**: This refers to rapid, shallow breathing.
- **Hyperpnoea**: This means panting.
- **Apnoea**: This means no breathing is taking place.
- **Cheyne-Stokes**: This is irregular breathing (deep breaths, then fast shallow breaths) seen shortly before death.
- **Dyspnoea**: This means difficulty breathing in or out and is often painful.

Signs of difficulty breathing include:

- Forced breathing out
- Flaring of nostrils
- Extended head and neck
- Elbows are rotated away from the chest
- Breathing through the mouth
- Exaggerated movements of the chest and abdomen
- Sounds
- Unable to settle

LIFE SAVING TECHNIQUES

- The heart has stopped – cardiac arrest
- The breathing has stopped – respiratory arrest

The two situations listed above are jointly referred to as cardio-pulmonary arrest (pulmonary is the term used for the vessels that take the blood to the lungs and back to the heart). The objective of cardio-pulmonary resuscitation is to restore heart and lung action and to prevent irreversible brain damage, which will occur if the tissues are deprived of oxygen for any length of time. Damage to body cells is thought to occur after 3–4 minutes following cardiac arrest. Therefore, it is important to be adequately prepared for the management of these emergencies and to recognise that time is short if permanent damage to body tissues is to be avoided.

> In veterinary practice resuscitation methods do include the use of drugs that stimulate the heart and the breathing, but these are administered only by a veterinary surgeon and therefore are not a first aid procedure.

Cardiac compression

Small dogs or cats

- Place the animal in recovery position (on its right side, head and neck extended, and tongue pulled forwards.
- Take hold of its chest between the thumb and fingers of the same hand over the heart and just behind the elbows.
- Support the body of the animal with the other hand on the lumbar spine area.
- At all times keep the head and neck in a straight line to assist breathing.
- Squeeze the thumb and fingers of the hand over the heart together, this will compress the chest wall and the heart which is squeezed between the ribs.
- Repeat this action approximately 120 times per minute.
- Keep a watch for the heart contractions re-starting.

Medium-sized dogs

- Place the animal in recovery position.
- Put the heel of one hand on the top of the chest, just behind the elbow and over the heart (Fig. 7.10).
- Place the other hand either on top of the first hand or under the animal to support the heart as it is compressed.
- Press down onto the chest with firm, sharp movements.
- Repeat this action about 80–100 times per minute.
- Keep a watch for the heart contractions re-starting.

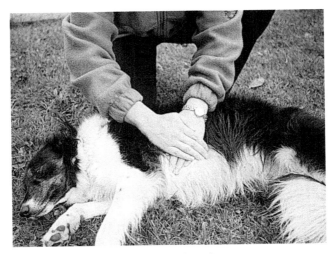

Fig. 7.10 Hand position for cardiac massage (medium dog).

Large, barrel-chested or fat dogs

- Place the animal on its back, with its head slightly lower than its body.
- Put the heel of one hand on the abdominal end of the sternum.
- Place the other hand on top of the first.
- Press firmly onto the chest, pushing the hands forwards towards the head of the animal.
- Keep the head and neck straight during the procedure at all times.
- Press down in this way for 80–100 times per minute.
- Keep a watch for the heart contractions re-starting.

Fig. 7.11 shows the hand position for cardiac massage for a large, non-barrel chested breed dog. Whatever the size of the animal, stop at 20-second intervals to check the heart beat or pulse and then continue.

Respiratory arrest

Whatever the cause, if the breathing has stopped then it must be urgently re-started. There are two methods for re-starting the breathing:

(1) Artificial respiration – manual method
(2) Mouth-to-nose technique

Artificial respiration

- Place in recovery position
- Clear airway of any blocking material
- Place a hand over the ribs, behind the shoulder bone (Fig. 7.12).

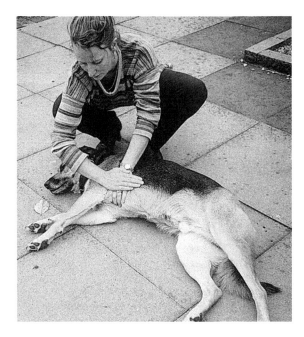

Fig. 7.11 Hand position for cardiac massage (large dog).

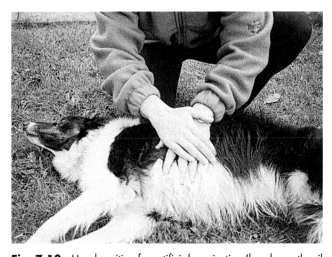

Fig. 7.12 Hand position for artificial respiration (hand over the ribs and behind the shoulder).

- Compress the chest with a sharp downward movement.
- Allow the chest to expand and then repeat the downward movement.
- The compressions are repeated at approximately 3–5-second intervals, until breathing re-starts.
- Keep head and neck straight at all times to assist airway.

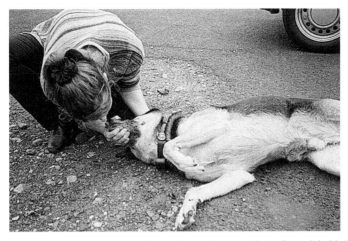

Fig. 7.13 Mouth-to-nose resuscitation with the airway kept straight and mouth held shut; the operator breathes down the nose.

Mouth-to-nose technique

- Place the animal in recovery position.
- Clear the airway.
- Place a tissue or thin cloth over the animal's nose (for personal safety).
- Hold the animal's neck straight at all times.
- Keep its mouth closed by holding the upper and lower jaws together.
- Breathe down its nose to inflate the lungs (Fig. 7.13).
- Repeat this at 3–5-second intervals.
- Keep a watch for the breathing re-starting.

This technique provides the animal with the unused oxygen in the handler's breath and their exhaled carbon dioxide, which help to stimulate the breathing reflex or gasp reflex in the animal.

BLEEDING (HAEMORRHAGE)

Bleeding or haemorrhage is the escape of blood from damaged blood vessels and can cause serious problems. Heavy bleeding can decrease the circulating blood volume enough to cause shock. Even small losses of blood over a period of time can potentially put the animal at risk.

Bleeding is not always visible; it may be internal, especially after a fall or road traffic accident. Therefore, look out for the general signs of bleeding:

- Colour – pale.
- Attitude – dull or listless.
- Appears thirsty.
- The pulse and breathing rate are fast and may appear feeble.

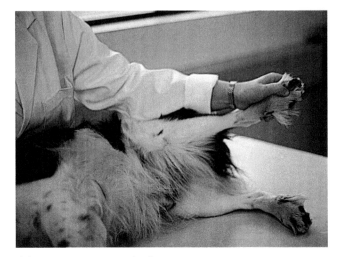

Fig. 7.14 Feel the extremities to assess body temperature.

- Feet and tail (extremities) are cold to touch (Fig. 7.14).
- Body temperature if taken is sub-normal.
- Capillary refill time is slow.

If blood loss is severe the signs will include those of reduced blood flow to vital organs such as:

- Animal becomes restless and will not settle
- It has difficulty breathing
- It may have fitting-type episode
- Animal unable to stand and becomes unconscious

Which blood vessel is damaged?

- **Artery**: The blood is bright red (oxygenated) in colour and comes out in spurts which are synchronised with the heart beat.
- **Vein**: The blood is dark red (de-oxygenated) in colour and it flows steadily.
- **Capillary**: The blood is bright red, involving small arteries and veins, and comes out as a steady ooze.

Methods of arresting bleeding

Whichever method is used, it must *not* interfere with the ability of the animal to breathe, preferably in a normal manner via the nose. Therefore, in the case of a nose bleed (epistaxis), while attempting to slow the blood loss no first aid treatment should interfere with the airway. The methods described below are meant for temporary relief and can be used for only a limited amount of time, until the veterinary surgeon takes over.

Digital or finger pressure

This method is used on a surface wound. A sterile or clean pad of absorbent material is pressed onto the area to control the blood loss. Care must be used with this method in case there is a piece of metal, glass or wood imbedded in the wound tissues, because pressing would push it deeper, and it would be harder to locate or may cause damage to internal structures. The time limit for this method is about 5–15 minutes after which the tissues beyond must receive a reviving flow of blood. After this the pressure can be applied again.

Pressure points

In several locations around the body, major arteries are positioned near the body surface, many passing over a solid structure such as bone. These tend to supply blood to the extremities, i.e. limbs and tail. Pressure on an artery where it crosses a bone can slow or even stop the blood supply reaching the area beyond. If the wound is on the extremity, these points can be used to apply pressure as a temporary measure to stop blood loss.

- Fore limbs – Pressure is put on the inside on the medial elbow area to slow the brachial artery (Fig. 7.15).
- Hind limbs – Pressure is put on the same site used for taking the pulse in the groin area on the femur to slow the femoral artery.
- Tail – Pressure is applied to the ventral or under-side of the base of the tail to slow the coccygeal artery.

The time limit for application of pressure in these locations is about 5–10 minutes. After this allow the blood flow to restore tissues. Re-application of pressure or use of another method may be required before the veterinary surgeon takes over.

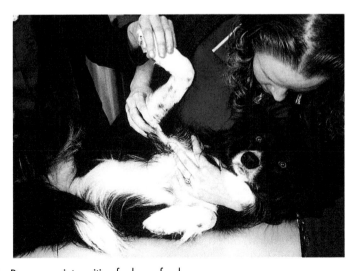

Fig. 7.15 Pressure point position for lower foreleg.

Pressure bandages

These may be used initially or after one or both of the previous methods have been used if the bleeding has not stopped prior to arrival of veterinary help. Pressure bandages can be applied only to extremities, i.e. the limbs (below elbow or knee) and tail. They are applied tightly to constrict and slow the blood flow in the surface vessels supplying the area, thus limiting blood loss.

The bandage is applied with plenty of padding material backing the dressing over the wound. It is tightly bandaged in place to include the foot area. If blood seeps through this bandage then more padding is applied and bandaged in place. If the foot is not included swelling will occur below the bandaged area due to the obstruction caused to the tissue fluid return to the trunk from the extremity. This is again only a temporary measure until arrival at the veterinary surgery. It can be put on for about an hour before the tissues must be released from the tight bandage and flow restored.

SHOCK

Shock is a term used to describe a complex and potentially fatal clinical syndrome which always involves insufficient blood to the tissues, with resulting lack of oxygen to the cells. This lack of oxygen to the cells is called tissue hypoxia and can be fatal if not corrected.

When blood is lost because of bleeding from a damaged blood vessel, the body tries to compensate by re-distributing blood to vital structures such as the brain and heart at the expense of other organs like the kidneys, skin, intestines and muscles. The resulting tissue hypoxia can cause severe damage to the organs.

There are various causes of shock. Some examples are:

• Blood loss from damaged vessels
• Pain or stress in highly strung animals
• Heart problems that interfere with the normal pumping action of the heart

The signs of shock include:

• Pale colour
• Cold extremities
• The animal becomes weak, slipping into an unconscious state
• Increase in the heart rate and breathing
• Slow capillary refill time of longer than 2 seconds

Until the animal can be treated by the veterinary surgeon, the handler must start the preventive shock procedure. Probably the single most useful thing that can be done is to maintain the body temperature. If the body is not allowed to shut down the surface (peripheral) blood vessels to the limbs and tail then established shock will at least be delayed, possibly even prevented.

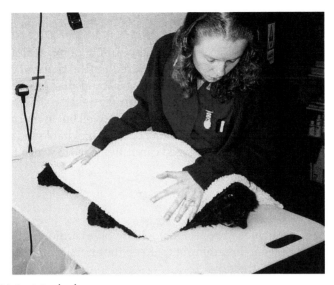

Fig. 7.16 Maintaining body temperature.

Shock has three forms:

(1) Impending: It is expected to happen bearing in mind the events or injuries suffered by the animal.
(2) Established: If it is in place, the animal must receive urgent medical treatment involving whole blood transfusion or use of plasma expanders.
(3) Irreversible: Treatment is unlikely to save the animal's life as the body systems are too severely damaged.

Treatment is aimed at not allowing shock to move on beyond the impending stage. To achieve this:

- Maintain the body temperature by wrapping the animal in blankets or towels (Fig. 7.16) and keep massaging or rubbing the extremities (feet and legs) to stimulate the blood flow. Never use artificial heat as the animal's temperature may get too high.
- Position the head slightly lower than the body to encourage the flow of blood to the brain.
- Stop any further blood loss.
- Help the animal to breathe by placing in recovery position, and if required give artificial respiration if breathing stops.
- Record the pulse.
- Transfer to the veterinary surgery as soon as possible.

HEART CONDITION

A correctly functioning heart is essential for the supply of oxygen, nutrients and other elements to all body cells. It is also required for the removal of waste and by-products from the body tissues. If anything should disrupt the function of the heart, the entire body is affected. Heart disease may develop slowly or may have been present from birth. Often the animal copes quite well but in the case of serious heart disease progression to heart failure may become inevitable and any stressful situation for that animal must be managed carefully. Signs to watch for are:

• Breathlessness
• Coughing after rest
• Fainting

Treatment (if the animal is unconscious) will involve cardio-pulmonary resuscitation if the heart beat and breathing stop. Keep the animal warm to avoid shock and seek veterinary help urgently.

POISONING

A poison or toxin is any substance, which on entry to the body in sufficient amounts, has a harmful effect on the individual concerned. Dogs are likely to eat almost anything and therefore become poisoned more frequently than cats. However, primary poisoning can also occur in a cat that has licked a poisonous substance attached to its coat. The cat has a poorly developed liver enzyme system for detoxification. Therefore the effects of poisoning can be very serious. Secondary poisoning can also occur in cats, in particular, after a cat has eaten baited mice, rats and other pests.

Poison can gain entry to the body by various means:

• Through the mouth (eaten or during self-grooming)
• Breathing in
• Absorption through the skin surface
• Through a cut

Animals can be poisoned by any of a multitude of potentially toxic substances, a lot of which are ordinary household products. The source may be poisonous plants or toxic chemicals including:

• Pesticides for the garden, e.g. slug bait, path clear, moss killer, etc.
• Rodent killers, e.g. warfarin
• Paint and cleaning solutions for brushes
• Disinfectants, e.g. bleach and toilet cleaners
• Drugs, e.g. aspirin, blood pressure tablets and sleeping tablets

Aspirin is a poison for cats since as a result of their metabolism the effect of this drug can last for up to 30 hours (approximately 12 hours in a dog), and this can lead to overdose if the owner re-medicates too soon. Cats can become poisoned when self-grooming, in particular from products such as paint brush cleaners, creosote-type paints and oils.

If a cat's coat hair is contaminated by any product, remove the contaminant as soon as possible, wearing gloves to avoid contact with the product on the coat. Use washing-up liquid on a *dry coat* and lubricate the affected hair area working the liquid soap with fingers into individual hair bundles until the contaminant starts to come away. Wash off with warm water and use a cat-approved shampoo on the now wet coat. Rinse thoroughly and dry the cat. Treat for shock and seek veterinary help if required. Do not use any liquid soap other than washing-up liquid (or cat-approved shampoo) which is produced sufficiently dilute to cause no harm to human hands, whereas detergents could act like a poison for the cat.

Very few poisons result in distinct signs. Most cause non-specific signs such that initially all that the owner notices is that the animal is behaving differently, and only later becoming aggressive, excited or depressed and/or unsteady on its feet, salivating, vomiting and or having diarrhoea, abdominal pain and fitting-type episodes. It may also be pale, have a lowered body temperature and slow capillary refill time.

The owner knows best about what is normal and what is unusual in their pet, therefore record all reported information and get in touch with the veterinary surgeon as soon as possible for advice on what to do next. If the owner knows which chemical was involved and has the container or packet take that to the veterinary surgery too. Unless instructed, do not make the animal sick, as this may cause more harm, particularly if the poison is corrosive. Until the veterinary surgeon takes over:

- Place the animal in recovery position.
- Provide support for any breathing problems.
- Keep it warm to reduce shock.
- Record pulse and heart rate.
- Comfort and do not leave unattended.
- Transfer to the veterinary surgery as soon as possible.

INSECT STINGS

Stings are usually more painful than they are harmful. However, it is possible that an animal may have an allergic reaction to the insect venom, or that the sting is close to the animal's airway and could obstruct breathing. If the venom sack is imbedded in the skin, never squeeze it as this may inject more venom into the animal. Remove carefully if possible, or leave it in place for the veterinary surgeon to remove in the safety of the practice.

- Wasp stings: These are alkaline. Treatment therefore consists of an acid solution like household vinegar in the form of a pad or compress.
- Bee stings: These are acidic. Treatment therefore consists of an alkaline such as bicarbonate of soda mixed with water and soaked into a pad or compress.

The aim of the treatment is to neutralise the situation. It is not always possible to know which insect is involved unless someone has seen the sting happen. If you are not sure what the insect was, apply a cold compress or face flannel filled with ice cubes to the area to reduce the swelling and give some pain control prior to any veterinary treatment.

FRACTURES

A fracture is a crack in the surface of a bone or a complete break in a bone. The objectives of first aid for fractures are to prevent the situation getting worse and to make the animal comfortable for safe transportation to a veterinary surgery. The causes of bones fracturing are varied and include:

- Road traffic accidents.
- The animal landing badly after jumping.
- Uncontrolled fall from a high surface or table.

Types of fracture

- Simple: The bone is broken but there is no connecting skin injury.
- Compound: The bone is broken and there is a wound connecting to the skin or the bone is protruding through the skin. A badly handled simple fracture can become a compound fracture.

Fig. 7.17 shows a fractured right femur and extent of tissue swelling. The signs of a fracture include:

- Loss of use of affected limb, which will not weight bear.
- Pain on handling, or the animal will not allow handling.

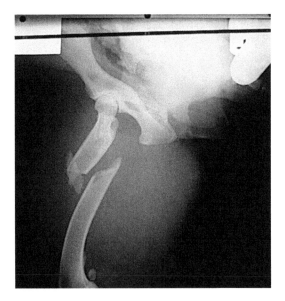

Fig. 7.17 X-ray of a fractured femur showing extent of tissue swelling.

- Unusual position, shape or movement of the limb.
- Swelling and bruising.

The best treatment for an animal with fractured bones is to get it to the veterinary surgery quickly, while taking care not to cause any further injuries by careless handling. Some fractures are also complicated by damage to other or surrounding tissues such as blood vessels, nerves or organs. Depending on the fracture, first aid consists of:

- Stopping any bleeding.
- Cleaning and covering any wounds.

Immobilise the fracture site if possible. This is only possible if the joints above and below the site can be immobilised by a splint. If splinting is possible, always apply the splint to the limb in the position in which it was found. For example, if the foot of the fore leg is positioned sideways instead of facing the front do not correct the position – splint it as you find it. Materials used for splinting are:

- Rolled-up magazine or newspaper
- Ruler or piece of wood

Which parts of the body can be splinted?

- Fore limb – from elbow to toes
- Hind limb – from stifle to toes
- Tail

If splinting is not possible:

- Confine the animal on plenty of bedding.
- Comfort and do not leave unattended.
- Treat for shock.
- Handle with care so as not to move the fracture unnecessarily.
- Take to the veterinary surgery urgently.

DISLOCATION

Dislocation is the displacement of one or more bones that form a joint. A dislocation differs from a fracture because displacement occurs only between joints and not along the length of a bone. Signs of a dislocation are similar to those of a fracture:

- Pain
- Abnormal joint function
- Shortening or lengthening of the limb involved
- Deformity and abnormal joint position or angle

The commonest simple dislocation involves the patella (knee cap). It can occur as a result of trauma in a road traffic accident, but it can also be a hereditary defect, particularly in small breeds of dog. Knee dislocation varies from very mild (an occasional medial slip of the patella) to very severe (the patella permanently out of position). A temporary limp is seen if the patella is capable of returning into the normal position after a dislocation. In this case on lifting the leg the patella will slip back into position and the leg can be placed back on the ground once more. If the patella is more permanently out of position:

- Do not attempt to place it back ino position.
- A cold compress on the knee may help with pain.
- Treat for shock.
- Seek veterinary help.

SOFT TISSUE INJURY

- **Sprain**: This always involves a joint with damage to the surrounding ligaments and other tissues. Recovery is slow as the torn and stretched tissue repairs. Common sites are fore and hind feet.
- **Strain**: This involves a muscle with tearing or stretching of the tissue. It can happen anywhere in the body; however, common sites are lower front leg, neck and shoulder muscles.

These injuries may require veterinary treatment depending on the amount of muscle damage, pain and inability to use the affected area.

WOUNDS

Wound refers to damage to the continuous structure of any tissue in the body, most commonly the surface of the skin.

Healing of wounds

Healing by first intention takes place in wounds that:

- Are not contaminated with grit, soil and micro-organisms.
- Have clean-cut edges that can be held together.
- Have been cleaned within one hour of injury.
- Heal, as the edges re-join, by 10 days after the injury.

Healing by second intention or granulation takes place in wounds that:

- Are contaminated with grit, soil and micro-organisms.
- Have jagged edges and possibly sections of skin missing.
- Have not been cleaned within two hours of injury.
- Have edges that gape open.

- Are infected.
- Take weeks or months to heal.

Wounds are described as being open or closed. A *closed wound* is one which does not penetrate the whole thickness of the skin, such as bruises or blood blisters (haematoma) or pockets of blood from a small damaged blood vessel. Treatment of these wounds involves use of a cold compress, such as ice cubes held in a face flannel, immediately after the injury to reduce the swelling of local tissues and help control pain. This treatment is useful only immediately after the injury.

Open wounds are those with damage to surface tissue and some bleeding. They are named according to the type of damage and whether or not tissue is missing:

- Incised wounds: These have clean-cut edges, are painful due to damage to the surface nerve endings and tend to bleed freely. They are caused by objects with sharp edges like scissors or a knife blade.
- Lacerated wounds: These have jagged flaps of skin, and sometimes skin sections are missing (avulsed). However because tissue is torn and stretched they are less painful than incised wounds and do not bleed much. They are caused by bite injuries, clippers or combs.
- Puncture wounds: These wounds have a long narrow tract going deep into the tissues, with only a small opening on the skin over the tract which is covered by scab. (Fig. 7.18). The scab traps microbes in the tract. The wound is caused by sharp-pointed objects like teeth (bite wounds) or scissors. They may also be caused by an in-growing toe nail or cork screw nail (although the tract is not that deep, these still provide a site for infection to develop). All such wounds are contaminated with the microbes trapped in the damaged tract. The microbes multiply, causing a localised infection to develop, which, if allowed to increase in size, becomes an abscess. Abscesses are very painful, often causing loss of limb function if located in the nearby tissues.

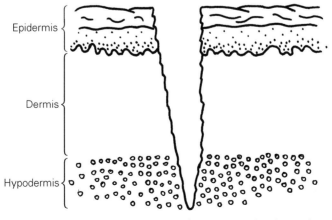

Fig. 7.18 Puncture wounds have a long narrow track and can lead to abscess formation.

- Abrasions and scratches: These are seen as bits of torn, ragged surface skin, with contaminants imbedded in the damaged areas. They are caused by friction and overheated or damaged clipper blades. The damage due to tearing is seen as oozing of serum from damaged capillaries in the surface layers of the skin only. These injuries are painful, bruised, and often inflamed.
- Fly strike (myiasis): This is seen when blow-flies lay eggs around the edges of an open wound. On hatching, the fly larvae crawl into the wound and burrow into the damaged tissues. The larvae feed on the wound fluids and living tissue, causing pain to the host animal. A reddish-brown fluid is usually seen on the coat hair and the area can be foul smelling.

Wound care

The sooner an open wound is cleaned using water-based antiseptic solution, the more chance there is that infection will not develop. **Solutions used for wound cleaning must not cause any further inflammation or damage to the wound, and therefore should not contain any soap or detergent**. Prevention of multiplication of micro-organisms in the wound can mean all the difference between the wound healing within ten days (first intention) and delayed healing (second intention or granulation).

First of all clip away the hair around the wound to expose the site, and then clean the area if possible. Solutions to use for cleaning are:

- Tap water
- Dilute antiseptic and water

Once the wound has been cleaned always cover it to prevent contamination and the animal aggravating the area further, and seek veterinary assistance.

EYE INJURIES

Any animal with eye injuries will have impaired sight and will be in pain. It is very important to approach the animal slowly and talk to it so that it is warned of your approach. The animal will be frightened and could injure the handler unless precautions are observed and correct handling techniques are used.

The types of injury seen include:

- Injuries caused by chemicals: These can cause serious injury to the eye structures. Always irrigate as soon as possible using tap water to remove any chemical. Do not leave unattended and seek medical help.
- Prolapsed eye ball: This means that the eye is now in front of the lids, and the optic nerve cord is being stretched as the lids swell. Never touch the eye ball. The treatment is as follows:
  - (a) Keep the eye moist at all costs. Use tap water soaked into a pad and squeeze onto the eye to moisten.

(b) Once moistened, soak the pad again in tap water and place gently over the eye.

(c) Hold or bandage in position.

(d) Do not leave unattended and stop any attempts at self-mutilation.

(e) Keep warm and quiet and treat for shock.

(f) Seek veterinary assistance urgently.

The important point to remember is that the eye must not be allowed to dry out. Some breeds of dog are prone to eye prolapse due to their short faces, such as Pug, Pekinese and Boxers. Therefore always use extra care when handling these breeds.

If the handler is present when the prolapse happens, return the eye to its place by holding the upper and lower eye lids and pulling them gently over the eye ball. This is possible only immediately after the injury. Do not attempt to do this if the eye has been prolapsed for longer than ten minutes and follow the above mentioned steps.

- Perforating injury: These are seen when a sharp object or instrument becomes imbedded in the structure of the eye. Never pull the foreign body out of the eye even if it is large enough to grasp. If it is removed non-surgically the fluid in the front chamber of the eye (aqueous humour) can leak, causing the back chamber to prolapse forward, thereby destroying the structure of the eye. Management involves keeping the eye moist (see eye prolapse above), preventing self-mutilation, and taking the animal to the veterinary surgery urgently.

PARAPHIMOSIS

Paraphimosis is the inability of an engorged penis to retract back into the prepuce following erection and or mating. Treatment is aimed at protecting the exposed penis, attempting to replace it into the prepuce. The animal may inadvertently self-mutilate this tissue further by licking. This causes considerable damage to the mucous membrane covering the penis followed by development of a substantial swelling. Keep the exposed tissue wet using water, as it is essential that the tissue is not allowed to become dry. Cold packs may be helpful in reducing the swelling sufficiently to replace the penis in the prepuce. Veterinary help must be sought if reduction is not possible by this method.

METABOLIC PROBLEMS

The following conditions can become first aid situations.

- Diabetes mellitus
- Epilepsy

Diabetes mellitus

There are several forms of the disease but they all cause the same problem, which is too much glucose in the blood. Diabetes is controlled by the animal's owner by (i) giving insulin injections, which moves the glucose out of the blood and into cells of the body, and (ii) controlling dietary intake to reduce glucose absorption from the intestine. These two actions help to reduce circulating blood glucose concentrations.

You should also be aware of the signs associated with low blood sugar (hypoglycaemia). This can occur in a diabetic animal when insulin is being given but the animal is not eating, resulting in an insulin overdose. At the same time, it is important not to allow the blood glucose to fall too low. This can be prevented by ensuring correct timing of feeding in relation to insulin administration.

Diabetic coma (hyperglycaemia) can develop if insulin has not been given, because of excess glucose in the blood. The signs of diabetic coma include:

- Lowered exercise tolerance
- Drowsiness
- Aggression
- Unwillingness to eat
- Staggering gait

These signs will be followed by muscle weakness, collapse and coma. If the animal becomes unconscious, oral glucose should not be given and the animal should be taken to a veterinary practice as quickly as possible.

Epilepsy

Epilepsy is also referred to as convulsion, fit or seizure. The animal appears to lose control of its body during a seizure-like episode. The cause is very difficult to determine due to the wide variety of occurrences and is linked to alteration of the electrical activity within the brain, which leads to loss of consciousness. Possible causes of epilepsy in animals include:

- Low blood sugar (hypoglycaemia)
- Stress in highly strung animals

Based on severity, epilepsy can be:

- Petit mal: This lasts a few seconds known as an absence, and it affects only a part of the brain. The signs include inattention, staring into space and apparent confusion.
- Grand mal: This is severe, lasting minutes to hours and affecting the entire brain. The animal is seen to have muscular twitches and contractions followed by a loss of consciousness, paddling of limbs, shivering and incontinence.
- Status epilepticus: This refers to repeated fitting episodes, one after another. The episode cannot be shortened by first aid but can be prolonged by continued stimulation from loud noises (radio, music or TV) bright lights or rough

handling. Therefore management of the situation is important to prevent other injuries occurring while the animal is convulsing.

Prior to examination by a veterinary surgeon, one should take note of the following:

- Do not attempt to restrain.
- Subdue light, reduce noise.
- Partly open a window or door for fresh air.
- Remove as many objects (e.g. furniture) as possible from the room or push them back out of the animal's way.
- Do not leave unattended for long and ensure that the airway is not obstructed (e.g. by vomit or its tongue).
- Only handle when the animal begins to recover, checking to see if it is able to respond to its name.

HEAT STROKE

A heat stroke results from an excessive rise in body temperature caused by high environmental temperatures. Dogs and cats do not lose body heat through the skin due to their dense coats and lack of sweat glands. Therefore to eliminate excess body heat they use the respiratory system, inhaling cool air through the nose and exhaling the hot air through the mouth. The faster this exchange occurs the faster their body will cool down – which is why dogs pant after exercise. The normal range of body temperature range is given earlier in the chapter.

Heat stroke is rarely seen in cats, and in dogs it usually occurs because the animal has been confined, on a hot day with no access to shade, in the drying area of a salon or in a car/vehicle with insufficient ventilation. **N.B. On a hot day the temperature in a car soon becomes higher than the environmental temperature even if windows are left open. Never leave an animal unattended in a car.**

When the environmental temperature exceeds the animal's body temperature it ultimately becomes impossible for that animal to maintain its body temperature within normal limits for that animal. Heat stroke affects all dogs, but most at risk if exposed to excess heat are:

- Those with thick dense coats
- Over-weight animals
- Short-nosed breeds
- Animals with heart conditions
- Elderly animals
- Those with medical conditions that affect breathing

In heat stroke, panting becomes ineffective and the body temperature rises rapidly, Death follows quickly if the body temperature is not immediately reduced. Signs of heat stroke include:

- Excess panting and salivation
- Bright red mucous membranes (check the gums)
- Vomiting
- Excitement/anxiety
- Disorientation
- Collapse/unable to stand
- High body temperature (41–43°C)

It is essential to reduce body temperature urgently as follows:

- Remove the animal from the hot environment.
- Cool it, using a pack of frozen vegetables held on the neck area.
- Wrap in towel/blanket soaked with cold water, and continue to hose water over the soaked wrapping, keeping clear of the face.
- Monitor the animal's body temperature.
- If it has collapsed, put in recovery position to assist breathing.
- If it is conscious, encourage it to drink small amounts of water continuously (if unrestricted the animal may swallow too much too fast and vomit).
- Treat for shock if the temperature goes below the normal temperature.
- Even if the body temperature is restored, it is essential to have the animal checked by a veterinary surgeon as soon as possible in case of a repeat rise in temperature.

BANDAGING

Reasons for bandaging include:

- Protection of a wound.
- Prevention of self-mutilation and interference.
- Support for soft tissues (muscle or ligament) in sprains and strains.
- Stopping bleeding (pressure bandage).
- Prevention of contamination.

Layers of a bandage

- Dressings: These are placed against the wound to provide a sterile contact material that will prevent further contamination of the site.
- Padding: This provides the means of absorption and padding, e.g. cotton wool (Fig. 7.19).
- Bandage: This secures the padding and dressing and protects them from the environment and the patient (Fig. 7.20).

The bandage must be comfortable. If the bandage is applied too tightly the animal will try to remove it or the surface tissues will be damaged by the animal's constant chewing and licking. The bandage prevents the animal from interfering with the area under the bandage and limits movement in the case of broken bones

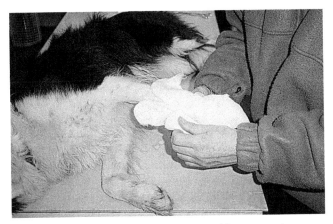

Fig. 7.19 The area to be bandaged is protected with a padding material.

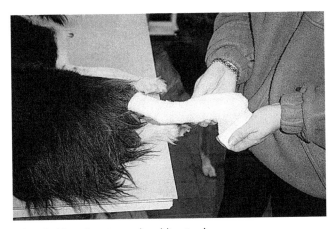

Fig. 7.20 Bandage holding dressing and padding in place.

or tissue damage, and therefore limits pain. The bandage should stay on for the required amount of time. Watch out for:

- Discomfort.
- Interference or self-mutilation (to try to remove the bandage).
- Bandage getting wet or dirty.

Rules for bandaging

- Wash hands before starting to prevent introducing infection.
- Collect all the materials together before restraining the animal.
- Never stick adhesive tape onto the animal's coat or hair, as it is hard to remove.
- Do not use safety pins or elastic bands to secure the ends of any bandage. Use narrow adhesive tape on the bandage surface.

- In the case of a leg bandage, include the foot otherwise it will swell.
- If unsure of the animal's temperament, muzzle for safety.

Applying a bandage

Limb bandage

It is important to apply the bandage in a spiral fashion (Fig. 7.21) to a leg to prevent development of pressure rings on the skin. A pressure ring forms when a bandage is applied in a circular manner or the bandage has slipped from its original position on the limb to lie as rings over one area.

A tight bandage can cause fluid to build up in the tissues, preventing it from flowing properly. To make sure a bandage is not applied too tightly, it should be possible to easily slip two fingers under the edge of the bandage (Fig. 7.22).

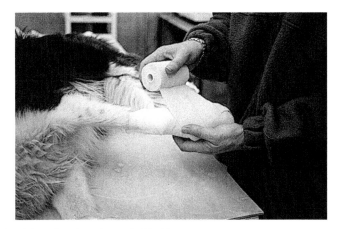

Fig. 7.21 Applying a bandage in a spiral fashion.

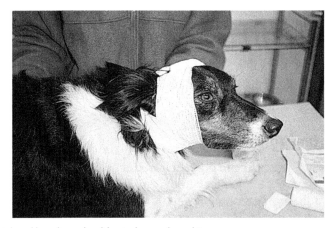

Fig. 7.22 A head bandage should not obstruct breathing.

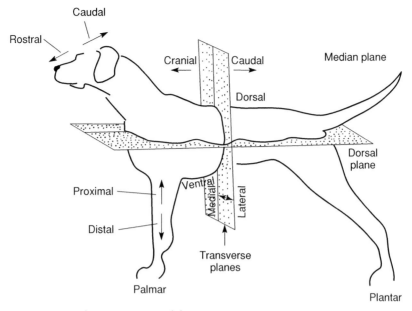

Fig. 7.23 Diagram showing anatomical directions.

ANATOMICAL DIRECTIONS

These are words in the language of medicine used for rapid communication for location of injury/or site description. Many of these words have originated from Greek or Latin, but are still in use today. Anatomical directions are used to describe areas of the animal's body and their direction and are useful if reporting an accident or injury case (Fig. 7.23).

The following four words are another way of saying above, below, front and back, respectively:

- Dorsal: Towards the top or the back surface of the body.
- Ventral: Towards the underside, below surface or nearer the ground.
- Cranial or anterior: Situated at the front of the body or towards the head end.
- Caudal or posterior: Situated towards the back end of the body or towards the tail.

Words that mean the side, middle of the body, or near the nose are:

- Lateral: To the side (left or right) or away from the middle of the body.
- Medial: The midline of a body structure or the body.
- Rostral: In the head but towards the nose.

Words that mean near or far from a named body structure (especially limbs) are:

- Proximal: Nearer to the body trunk or closer to a named structure.
- Distal: Away from the body trunk or further from a named structure.

Words which indicate the surface of a limb, especially the lower limb surfaces are:

- Palmar: Also called volar, indicating the caudal or back surface of the forelimb, below the carpus or wrist area.
- Plantar: Indicating the caudal or back surface of the hind limb, below the tarsus or hock area.

Words meaning inside or outside the body are:

- Internal: Inside the body.
- External: Outside or surface of the body.

Infectious Diseases in Dogs and Cats

Disease is defined as an abnormality of structure or function of a part of an organ or tissue in the body and is accompanied by a set of symptoms or behavioural changes in the affected animal. Infectious disease spreads from one animal to another by various methods. It is hard to know which organism is responsible in a particular case.

MICRO-ORGANISMS AND DISEASE

Micro-organisms live either in or on the body:

- Oral, nasal and eye discharge
- Urine
- Vomit
- Blood
- Skin surface

Sometimes the disease is passed on by a 'carrier' animal. These animals do not show clinical signs of disease but:

- May have had the disease and recovered – convalescent carriers.
- May never show clinical signs of the disease – healthy carriers.

Both types of carrier will shed the disease-carrying micro-organism into their environment, putting other animals at risk. Thus, micro-organisms are passed by:

- Direct contact: When parts of the bodies of two animals come into contact, e.g. nose to nose or nose to anus.
- Indirect contact: The contact is an inanimate object, e.g. bedding, water bowl or lamp post.
- Aerosol transmission: This occurs through the air, in the form of droplets from sneezing, coughing, or using air currents.
- Contaminated food or water: When these have been contaminated by urine and faeces of passing rodents or others.

- Carrier animals: These shed microbes in discharge, urine or faeces although unaffected themselves, e.g. canine hepatitis.

Incubation

Incubation is the time between the animal receiving the microbe and showing clinical signs of disease. The incubation time depends on:

- Quantity of microbes: If the microbes enter via the respiratory and/or digestive tract, the secretions will decrease the ability of the disease to spread unless the animal is susceptible (see next point).
- Immune status of the animal: If an adequate immune response is not possible the microbes will overcome the host animal's resistance.
- General health: If this is not good then the animal is possibly susceptible.
- Age: The immune response of the body is affected in very young and old animals.

Infection

If the micro-organism has entered the host animal and overcome its resistance, infection may ensue. Some infections are confined to a restricted area, e.g. abscesses, whereas others are termed 'systemic' because they spread through the whole body via the bloodstream.

> **Terms related to infections**
> - Clinical infection: Signs of infection are observed
> - Subclinical infection: No clinical signs present
> - Bacteraemia: Bacteria are present in the bloodstream
> - Septicaemia: Bacteria are multiplying in the bloodstream

METHODS OF DISEASE CONTROL

- Avoid direct contact between infected and healthy animals.
- Maintain high levels of hygiene/disinfection in the animal's environment.
- Provide treatment for the infected animal.
- Control parasites to prevent disease passing to healthy animals.
- Maintain vaccination status.

Bacteria

Bacteria are single-celled organisms. Most are large enough to be seen using a light microscope. Their size and shape (Fig. 8.1) can vary which helps in their classification. In favourable conditions bacteria reproduce by dividing into two

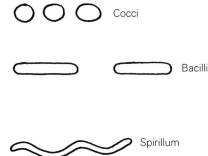

Fig. 8.1 Bacterial shapes.

every 15–20 minutes (binary fission). In conditions unfavourable for growth some bacteria will form spores with a protective surrounding wall. The bacteria can remain inside the spores for many years. Passing on of genetic material and information from a bacterial donor to a recipient bacterium is called conjugation and is a method of survival of bacteria.

Viruses

Viruses are the smallest of the microbes. They are always parasitic, and reproduce by replicating themselves. This process happens after the viral DNA or RNA (genetic information) has gained entry into a living host (the cells in the animal's body). Different viruses target different types of body cell.

The viral strand of material takes over control of the host cell's metabolism and directs it to manufacture replicas of the viral material. When enough replicas have been produced, the virus will instruct the host cell to rupture, releasing the viruses, each of which can then use other host cells for the purpose of replicating.

The virus is not a cell – it consists of a protein coat around a DNA or RNA strand. Some viruses (Fig. 8.2) are also surrounded by a membrane known as an envelope, which may have structures like spikes on its surface for attaching to the host cell before entry.

In many cases, the cycle of viral replication causes no apparent harm to the host. Disease occurs when large numbers of host cells in a specific tissue are destroyed leading to disruption of body functions.

Fungi

These are non-chlorophyll-bearing plants. Fungi are divided into:

- Moulds (multi-cellular)
- Yeasts (uni-cellular)

Fungi do not have the ability to make their own food, and so must exist as parasites or saprophytes. Spread is by spores (Fig. 8.3). Reproduction in fungi is sexual (hyphae from different strains unite to form a survival spore, awaiting favourable conditions for growth). There is also an asexual method (spread of spores).

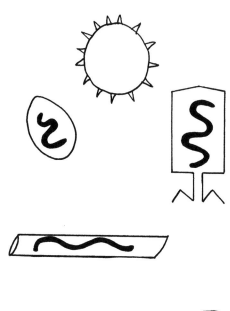

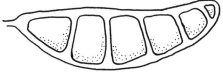

Fig. 8.2 Virus shapes showing DNA strand and protein coat.

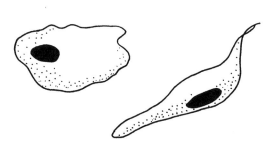

Fig. 8.3 Spindle-shaped cells make up the fungal spore, as seen in *Microsporum canine* (ringworm).

Fig. 8.4 Protozoal shapes. Protozoa are capable of changing shape for engulfing food particles.

Protozoa

These are single-celled animals and range in size from microscopic to just visible to the naked eye (Fig. 8.4). They have a cell membrane and organelles for move-ment (flagella and cilia). Reproduction is asexual by binary fission and nutrition is holozoic (capture and assimilation of organic material in their environment). They are capable of pursuing prey by following the trail of a chemical or are stimu-lated by movement. They are often found in water. Protozoa form cysts at some point in their life cycle. This is the form which passes from host to host, and allows survival outside the host temporarily.

Disease-causing micro-organisms

Microbe	Dog	Cat
Protozoa	Coccidiosis	Coccidiosis
	Toxoplasmosis	Toxoplasmosis
Fungal	Ringworm	Ringworm
Bacterial	Kennel cough	
	Leptospirosis	
Viral	Distemper	Panleucopenia
	Infectious hepatitis	Respiratory disease
	Parvovirus	Infectious peritonitis
		Leukaemia
		Immunodeficiency
	Rabies	Rabies

ZOONOSES

Zoonoses are diseases that are transmitted from animals to people. The disease in humans is frequently given a different name or described by symptoms only.

Disease in animals	Disease in humans
Leptospirosis	Weil's disease
Toxocariasis	Visceral larval migrans
Echinococcosis	Hydatid disease (hydatidosis)
Sarcoptic mange	Skin rash and bites
Cheyletiella mite	Parasite bite
Ringworm (dermatophyte)	Ringworm (dermatophyte or mycosis)
Salmonellosis	Salmonellosis
Rabies	Rabies (hydrophobia)

Examples of symptoms of zoonotic diseases are shown below.

Human disease	Signs
Pasteurellosis	Bites or scratches; become infected
Cat scratch fever	High temperature; 'flu-like signs; rash
Ringworm	Raised circular inflamed skin lesion
Toxoplasmosis	Abortion of fetus
Rabies	Fever; itching in the original bite area; behaviour change; paralysis and death

To minimise the risk to people of zoonoses passed by a dog or cat, the following simple but effective hygiene precautions are recommended to be taken in the grooming salon:

- Vaccination certificates should be checked prior to admitting animal to a salon and recorded on owner record.
- Recommend investigation to owner if any signs of illness observed and do not proceed with grooming.
- Recommend flea and worm control to owner
- Wash hands after handling any animal
- Always wear gloves when handling body discharge

DISEASES OF DOGS

Infectious canine diseases for which there is a vaccine include:

- Canine distemper
- Canine viral hepatitis
- Canine leptospirosis
- Canine parvovirus
- Canine infectious tracheobronchitis (kennel cough syndrome)
- Rabies

Canine distemper

The virus causing distemper attacks the following body systems:

- Central nervous system
- Respiratory system
- Gastrointestinal system
- Skin

The disease is caused by a paramyxovirus that is closely related to the measles virus of humans. The virus is inactivated by light, heat and most disinfectants. Distemper is commonly seen in 4–5-month-old puppies when no longer covered by maternal immunity. Distemper follows a seasonal occurrence (autumn and winter), due in part to the ability of the virus to survive in cold weather. The routes of infection are:

- Respiratory tract due to aerosol (airborne) exposure
- Mouth and eye mucous membranes

During the incubation period of 3–10 days, the virus replicates and travels via the lymphatic system to the lymph nodes, spleen, thymus and bone marrow. When the virus is in the lymph nodes, the body temperature rises to between 39°C and 40°C for 2–4 days. About half of all puppies infected are capable of mounting an adequate response and produce antibodies to clear the infection at this point. However, if the virus survives, it replicates in the epithelium, other organs and central nervous system. This allows secondary infection to occur. Clinical signs of distemper include:

- Lack of appetite (anorexia)
- Nasal and eye discharge
- Coughing
- Diarrhoea and vomiting
- Hardening of the footpads
- Inco-ordination
- Paralysis
- Epileptic-type fits

If the puppy survives the respiratory or gastrointestinal stage of the disease, it will develop neurological signs up to four weeks later. Older dogs tend to present with just the neurological signs. This stage is usually fatal; occasionally the dog will survive but there will be lasting central nervous system damage.

Vaccination gives good protection but is not life-long, so booster vaccinations are essential.

Canine infectious tracheobronchitis (kennel cough syndrome)

This syndrome is a complex disease linked to a number of viruses. The micro-organisms causing kennel cough syndrome include:

- *Bordetella bronchiseptica*
- Canine adenovirus type 2 (CAV2)
- Canine parainfluenza virus (CPIV)
- Canine distemper virus (CDV)

However, the major cause is thought to be the bacterium *Bordetella bronchiseptica*. Clinically the syndrome presents as tracheitis, which is usually self-limiting but which may also develop into bronchitis or pneumonia. *Bordetella bronchiseptica*, CAV2 and CPIV are highly contagious and commonly present when dogs are housed together, as they infect the respiratory tracts of dogs of any age. They cause nasal and tracheal inflammation lasting 5–14 days and then normally resolve, with the dog making a good recovery. At this time the dog sheds the organisms in respiratory secretions. Clinical signs of kennel cough syndrome include:

- Cough
- Sneezing and nasal discharge
- Depressed but still eating
- Retching after coughing

Transmission from dog to dog can be minimised by isolation of the affected animal and by improving kennel ventilation and disinfection routines. All dogs that are going into a boarding establishment should be vaccinated with a mixed vaccine that includes CAV2 and CPIV.

Canine parvovirus

The canine parvovirus is closely related to the feline panleucopenia virus. The virus is highly resistant to inactivation by most disinfectants except bleach and formalin-based chemicals and can survive for months in the environment. The virus localises in lymphatic tissues and the lining of the intestinal epithelium. It is found in vast numbers in the faeces and vomit of infected animals and causes myocarditis and mild to severe haemorrhagic enteritis.

The infection spreads by faecal or oral contact. Damage to the bone marrow results in lack of white cells and the infection spreads from lymph cells in the gut tissues. The incubation period is 5–10 days. Clinical signs of canine parvovirus infection include:

- Dull and depressed
- Anorexia
- High temperature (up to 41°C)
- Vomiting
- Bloodstained gastric juices
- Bloodstained diarrhoea 24 hours later
- Rapid dehydration

Vaccination as a puppy should be followed by annual boosters for protection.

Canine viral hepatitis

This is caused by the canine adenovirus type 1 (CAV1). Transmission occurs through oral and nasal passages after exposure to infected materials. The virus is resistant and survives outside the body for up to 11 days in bedding, feeding bowls, urine and faeces. It is resistant to freezing, ultraviolet light and most disinfectants but is destroyed by heat. Following exposure, the virus localises in the tonsils and lymph nodes where primary replication occurs. The virus travels in the lymph and gains access to the bloodstream. It is attracted to the cells of the liver and kidneys, where further replication occurs, before it is shed in urine and faeces. The incubation period is 5–9 days. Animals can shed the virus for several months after recovery.

Puppies may develop high temperature and death occurs within hours. Older dogs survive the viraemic stage but may have blood-stained vomit and diarrhoea, and acute abdominal pain. In some dogs, 'blue eye', clouding of the cornea of the eye, can occur up to three weeks after acute infection. Vaccination and annual boosters are essential.

Leptospirosis

Leptospirosis is also known as Stuttgart disease or Weil's disease in humans and is caused by a filament-like bacterium, *Leptospira icterohaemorrhagiae*, which causes a zoonotic disease in humans. *Leptospira* strains that cause the disease in dogs are:

- *Leptospira icterohaemorrhagiae*: Primary host is the rat, attacks mainly the liver.
- *Leptospira canicola*: Primary host is the dog, attacks mainly the kidney.

These bacteria are easily destroyed by sunlight, disinfectants and temperature extremes. The disease spreads by direct contact, bite wounds or ingestion of infected food or water. Rodents such as rats are frequently carriers, shedding the bacteria in urine and thus contaminating water. The incubation period is 7–21 days, with severity of the disease depending on the susceptibility of the host animal and the strain. Clinical signs of leptospirosis include:

- High temperature
- Shivering and muscle pain
- Vomiting and diarrhoea
- Dehydration
- Shock
- Jaundice (mucous membranes of mouth and eye appear yellow)

Animals continue to shed the bacteria via the urine for some time after recovery. Strict isolation must be observed. Both veterinary surgeon and doctor can provide advice and information regarding how to prevent a human carer becoming infected. An annual booster after initial vaccination is essential.

Rabies

Rabies is caused by a rhabdo virus. The virus is fragile, surviving for only a short time in the environment, and is destroyed by most disinfectants, heat and light.

It is transmitted in the saliva of infected animals, and replicates in the muscle cells at the site of infection. Then it travels via the peripheral nerves to the spinal cord and the brain. When it has invaded the central nervous tissues, neurological signs are observed. The virus also travels to the salivary glands, where it is shed to infect other mammals, both human and animal. Rabies is therefore a zoonotic disease.

The incubation period ranges from 10 days to four months, the time depending on how close to the central nervous system the virus initially enters the host. There are three phases or stages of the disease. However, all will not necessarily occur in all affected animals.

(1) Preclinical stage: This lasts 2–3 days. There is a raised body temperature, slow eye reflexes and signs of irritation at the site of the original injury.
(2) Excitable stage: This lasts up to one week with the animal becoming irritable, aggressive and disorientated, having difficulty standing and epileptic-type fits.
(3) Dumb stage: This lasts 2–4 days during which the animal's throat and skeletal muscles becomes progressively paralysed, leading to salivation, difficulty breathing, coma and death.

In some cases the preclinical stage can last for several months during which the virus is shed in the saliva. The diagnosis is confirmed on post-mortem examination of the brain and spinal cord for signs of the virus. A vaccine is available for dogs that live in countries where rabies is endemic or in case of travelling to a country with rabies in the wild or domestic animal population. The vaccine is given at three months of age with annual boosters.

If a human is bitten by an animal suspected of having rabies, the wound should be cleaned immediately using soap or antiseptic solution and medical attention should be sought straight away.

DISEASES OF CATS

Infectious feline diseases include:

- Rabies (see Rabies in the dog above)
- Feline leukaemia
- Feline panleucopenia or feline infectious enteritis
- Chlamydiosis or feline pneumonitis
- Feline viral respiratory disease:
  (a) Feline herpesvirus
  (b) Feline calicivirus
- Feline infectious anaemia
- Feline infectious peritonitis
- Feline immunodeficiency

Feline leukaemia

The retrovirus causing feline leukaemia (FLV) affects approximately 2% of cats worldwide. It is contagious and, once symptoms appear, almost always fatal. Most cats are exposed to this virus during their life and it is most commonly found where cats are in close contact.

Evidence of the virus is obtained from testing blood samples using the FLV enzyme-linked immunosorbent assay (ELISA) test. The effect of the virus on the host cat depends on the age of the cat when it is infected and the quantity of virus received.

Some cats become ill and apparently recover whereas others do not become ill and develop immunity to the disease. Yet others develop the disease symptoms after an incubation period of weeks to several years. Young kittens are most susceptible to the virus. Most die within 2–3 years of exposure or as a result of FLV-related conditions including anaemia (lack of red blood cells) and lymphosarcoma (tumours of the lymph system). Clinical signs of FLV include:

- High temperature
- Vomiting and diarrhoea
- Weight loss
- Kidney disease
- Enlargement of the spleen

The virus is shed in:

- Saliva
- Faeces
- Urine
- Milk to offspring

The virus is easily destroyed by disinfectants and cannot live long outside a host. Infection can be passed via saliva in bite/fight episodes, contact with other cats or from the mother to the kittens before or after birth via the milk. Initially, the virus replicates in the lymphatic tissues, then moves on to target other systems containing lymphatic tissue, such as the intestines, causing enteritis, the salivary glands and the urinary and reproductive systems, causing infertility or abortion in pregnant animals. The disease is controlled by:

- Testing. Testing for evidence of microbes in other cats in a multi-cat household may need to be done several times to confirm the result because the cat is euthanised if it is a true result.
- Isolating animals testing positive.
- Disinfection and maintenance of hygiene in cat areas.
- Re-testing 12 weeks after positive test to ensure result is correct.
- Testing all new cats that join a household.

After two positive tests, the safe option is to permanently isolate the infected cat or perform euthanasia. Cats are vaccinated from nine weeks of age with a second dose 2–4 weeks later followed by an annual booster. Before vaccination, all cats are tested for presence of the virus in the blood.

Feline panleucopenia or feline infectious enteritis

Feline panleucopenia is a highly infectious disease of cats. It is also known as:

- Feline parvovirus
- Feline distemper
- Feline infectious enteritis

The disease is caused by a parvovirus, similar to the canine parvovirus. The disease can affect cats of any age and is mainly responsible for deaths in young kittens. The virus is stable and capable of surviving in the environment for months to years and is resistant to most disinfectants. The incubation period is 2–10 days following direct contact with an infected animal or ingestion of the virus. The virus targets rapidly dividing cells and tissues of the small intestines, lymph and bone marrow. It is shed in saliva, vomit, faeces and urine. Clinical signs of infection with the feline parovirus include:

- Diarrhoea, often bloodstained
- Dull and listless behaviour
- Abdominal pain
- Fever and dehydration

Blood tests show a typical reduction in white blood cells (leucopenia), particularly neutrophils. The virus can cross the placenta during pregnancy and affects the fetus by targeting the brain tissue (cerebellum), causing death or abnormal nervous system development. Affected kittens show balance difficulties and incoordination at about 2–3 weeks of age. If the cat survives the first week of clinical disease, careful nursing can lead to recovery but the intestine may suffer permanent damage, evident as poor absorption of nutrients and frequent diarrhoeal episodes. Vaccination, using either live or inactivated vaccine (in pregnant cats), provides good immunity with a booster required every 1–2 years.

Chlamydiosis or feline pneumonitis

Chlamydial infection is caused by an organism which lives within cells. *Chlamydia* are therefore treated like a virus, although in appearance they resemble bacteria. *Chlamydia cati* or *C. psittaci* affects the conjunctiva of the eye in cats, causing severe conjunctivitis with eye discharge, sneezing and nasal discharge. The conjunctivitis may affect one or both eyes. Transmission is thought to be via contact with eye/nose discharge, or genital or gastrointestinal secretions from carrier animals. The incubation period is 3–10 days. Clinical signs of chlamydiosis include:

- Initial watery discharge in one eye, spreading to both
- Inflamed conjunctiva
- Fever
- Rubbing eyes and signs of discomfort
- Diarrhoea in kittens

During pregnancy, chlamydiosis may lead to abortion or stillbirth. Chlamydiosis may last for 2–3 weeks or longer, especially as a part of the feline viral respiratory disease complex. Animals may shed the responsible organism for several weeks so any treatment given usually continues for three weeks after recovery. The organism is killed by most disinfectants during routine cleaning. Vaccination is available with annual boosters.

Feline viral respiratory disease

This is also known as:

- Cat flu
- Feline upper respiratory disease (FURD)
- Feline viral rhinotracheitis (FVR)

The two main viruses involved are:

- Feline herpesvirus
- Feline calicivirus

Cats are particularly susceptible to infections (both bacterial and viral) of the nose and throat. Due to their location, these infections are called upper respiratory infections or cat 'flu. While it is essential to vaccinate, as with the 'human flu', vaccines do not protect against some strains of this disease, especially feline calicivirus.

Calicivirus is easily destroyed outside the host by disinfectants. Transmission of the virus is by aerosol or direct contact. As a result of this, any grouping of cats may lead to infection, e.g. shows, boarding, breeding kennels and veterinary surgeries. Many cats that survive the infection become carriers, shedding the virus for several years. It is possible to have suspected carrier animals tested by a veterinary surgeon for the presence of the calicivirus. The incubation period is up to ten days after exposure to high-risk situations (groups of cats) or stress caused by a change in the environment which may lower the cat's resistance. Clinical signs of the infection include:

- Ulcers on the tongue
- Inflammation of the gums
- Unwilling to eat, but producing excess saliva
- High temperature
- Depressed and listless
- Loss of voice

The presence of ulcers may allow bacteria normally present to add to the cat's original symptoms and recovery time.

Feline herpesvirus can survive outside the host for up to eight days. This virus attacks and replicates in the tissues of the respiratory tract and conjunctiva of the eye, causing viral rhinotracheitis. The tissues from the nose (rhino) to the trachea (tracheitis) are affected and inflamed, causing breathing difficulties, sneezing and coughing. Animals can act as carriers after recovering from the infection, shedding the virus particularly when stressed.

Viral rhinotracheitis is the most serious form of upper respiratory disease, often leaving animals after recovery with damage to the nasal passages. This causes the affected cat to periodically sneeze, snuffle and have a runny nose, the discharge occasionally being thick with pus. The incubation period lasts for 2–10 days following exposure. Clinical signs of the infection include:

- High temperature
- Discharge from eyes and nose, later becoming thickened due to bacterial infection
- Depressed and listless
- Loss of appetite
- Sneezing
- Conjunctivitis
- Mouth ulcers
- Pneumonia
- Abortion in pregnant queens

A vaccine is available, requiring an annual booster. It is administered intranasally. In high-risk situations, six-monthly administration is advisable.

Feline infectious anaemia

Infectious anaemia is the direct loss of red blood cells caused by a blood parasite called *Haemobartonella felis* or *Eperythrozoon felis*. It is thought to be transmitted via blood-sucking parasites, e.g. the flea. Cats of all ages can be affected. When the disease is linked to feline leukaemia, affecting white blood cell numbers, chances of recovery are poor.

The single-celled parasite responsible for the infection can be demonstrated on a blood smear in the laboratory. Discussion with a veterinary surgeon is essential at this time. Products to safely remove fleas from the affected household will be required and other cats in the same household may need to be examined and treated. The incubation period is up to 50 days, with recovered or carrier animals often shedding the parasite for months. Clinical signs of the infection include:

- Pale mucous membranes (mouth and gums)
- Breathing difficulty
- Listless and loss of appetite
- Third eyelid up as a sign of ill health
- High temperature
- Weight loss

Animals respond well to treatment using specific antibiotics. There is no vaccine against this virus.

Feline infectious peritonitis

Infectious peritonitis is also called feline infectious vasculitis and is caused by a coronavirus which affects mostly young cats under three years of age. It causes the lining membrane of the abdomen (peritoneum) and contents to become inflamed (peritonitis). The effects of this disease are not limited to the organs of the abdomen and it may also affect the nervous system and eyes.

One mode of transmission is contact between cats via urine and faeces. Carrier animals may carry the virus for years, with mothers possibly passing the disease to their kittens. The virus is unstable outside the body and easily destroyed by disinfectants. Diseased cats are sometimes affected by feline leukaemia, which may make them susceptible to the peritonitis virus. The form taken by the disease will vary depending on the ability of the animal's immune system to mount a response to the viral challenge. Clinical signs of the disease include:

- Lack of appetite and gradual weight loss
- Fever
- Swollen abdomen due to fluid accumulation
- Diarrhoea and vomiting

Later signs include:

- Organ failure
- Neurological signs including inability to stand, paralysis and convulsions
- Inflammation within the structure of the eye, affecting the sight

Depending on the form taken by the disease, it is often further described as *wet* (fluid in body cavities) or *dry* (tumour-like masses called granulomatous lesions forming in organs). The disease is controlled by observing strict hygiene measures and disinfection particularly in multi-cat households or where groups of cats are housed. There is no vaccine available in the UK at present.

Feline immunodeficiency

Feline immunodeficiency is caused by a virus of the lentivirus group. The disease is often characterised by a long incubation period from four weeks to several years; as a result, it is unusual to find the infection in cats under two years of age. The disease attacks the lymph system, causing the body's immune response to be suppressed. Initially the disease was known as T-lymphotrophic T cell lentivirus, due to the effect on the cells of the immune system (T cells and B cells).

The virus is carried in the saliva of the infected animal and transmitted by bite. Therefore cats that have access to outdoor life are more at risk than those living completely indoors. Male cats are more commonly infected due to territorial fighting.

Commercial screening kits are available for detection of antibodies to the virus in a blood sample from the animal. After the initial response to the virus, the cat shows signs of the disease in a few weeks. These signs are very similar to those of feline leukaemia and include:

- Conjunctivitis and nasal discharge
- Enlarged superficial lymph nodes (lymphadenopathy)
- Mouth and gum inflammation
- Diarrhoea
- Skin problems
- High temperature
- Neurological signs that include difficulty in walking and change in temperament

The animal then appears to recover but due to gradual suppression of its immune responses, it will frequently suffer from recurrent or ongoing infections of various kinds, often failing to respond to veterinary treatment. The cat will suffer weight loss, becoming inactive and listless. There is no vaccine available so owners are advised to castrate male cats and limit exposure to other neighbourhood cats to avoid contact with an infected animal.

IMMUNITY

Immunity is the body's natural protection against life-threatening diseases. Immunity may be acquired by passive or active means.

Passive immunity results from the transfer of maternal antibodies to the newborn via the colostrum and the milk. The degree of passive immunity depends on the quantity of the colostrum and the quality of the mother's own antibodies resulting from her recent vaccinations. Passive immunity lasts only as long as the antibodies remain active in the blood – from three to 12 weeks. After this time the body eliminates the antibodies.

Active immunity develops as a result of either the animal becoming infected with a micro-organism, developing the disease and recovering or by vaccination. Both cause the body to react in much the same manner by stimulating the production of antibodies, which are specific for particular microbes (pathogens or antigens).

The purpose of vaccination is to prevent the disease by averting or limiting the infection in a host animal. Vaccines stimulate the immune system, which in turn produces antibodies. The cells of the immune system responsible for producing this protection are the B lymphocytes (B cells) and these in turn are assisted by the T lymphocytes (T cells). Both are white blood cells, which may be targeted and destroyed by certain viruses. Antibodies recognise specific viruses or bacteria and prevent or limit their ability to produce disease in the host animal. Vaccines are prepared from live or inactivated (killed) preparations of micro-organisms.

At the time of vaccination, the veterinary surgeon will fully examine the animal to ensure that adverse conditions which may influence the manner in which the body responds to the vaccine are not present, such as a raised body temperature. Many factors influence an animal's ability to respond to vaccination. These include:

- Antibodies from the mother's milk which could interfere with the vaccine.
- Type of vaccine.
- Route of administration (subcutaneous or intranasal).
- Animal's age.
- Medication that could interfere with the vaccine, e.g. anti-inflammatory drugs.
- Diet.
- Infection already present.

Part 2
Getting Started

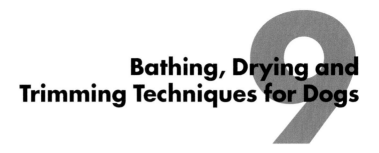

Bathing, Drying and
Trimming Techniques for Dogs

SMOOTH COAT

Breed example: Boxer (Wo-Sm)

Wash the coat with the appropriate shampoo for the skin type following the bathing routine described in Chapter 6. Ensure that you massage the shampoo thoroughly into the skin to remove any dead coat – a rubber brush can help with this.

Dry the dog with a moisture absorbent cloth, towel dry and use the blaster to remove any excess coat. If a cabinet dryer is available then finish drying the dog in there or use a stand dryer or hand dryer to ensure total dryness. Check that all the areas are thoroughly dry and then polish the coat with protein spray and a silk cloth or rubber brush.

DOUBLE COAT – TYPE ONE

Breed example: German Shepherd (Pa-Dc1)

This coat type can take a long time to bath if done thoroughly and correctly. Use a blaster first to remove dead undercoat and some dirt; this also opens the coat, allowing the shampoo to penetrate. Apply a good cleansing shampoo following the bathing routine described in Chapter 6. Use your fingers to work the shampoo deeply into the coat. A shampoo brush is also useful. Rinse thoroughly. If the dog has a lot of dead undercoat and tangles, apply conditioner and blast while the conditioner is in the coat. This enables the conditioner to sink into the coat and makes the drying process easier. It is vitally important to rinse thoroughly as shampoo or conditioner residue will make the coat dull and greasy.

To dry the coat, squeeze out any excess water from the coat with a moisture absorbent cloth. Use the blaster to remove the remaining water and undercoat. Towel dry. Use a drying cabinet if you have one available but remove the dog after ten minutes and blast again. If the coat is still very wet return the dog to the cabinet for five minutes but if it is not finish drying the coat with a stand dryer or hand-held dryer. Use a slicker brush and wide toothcomb to ensure removal of all dead undercoat.

DOUBLE COAT – TYPE TWO

Breed example: Bearded Collie (Pa-Dc2)

For a type two double coat use an all-purpose shampoo but if the coat is long and natural, do not rub too vigorously as this will cause tangles. Bath and apply shampoo following the coat growth. Brush through with a shampoo brush but if there are knots in the coat separate them with your fingers. Quite often, knots are more easily removed from a clean coat instead of battling through dirt and twigs! After rinsing, apply a good-quality conditioner. If the coat is out of condition or knotty, allow the conditioner to soak for five or ten minutes keeping the dog warm by wrapping it in a towel. Rinse thoroughly. Do not use a blaster on long coats as this will cause tangles.

For long-coated breeds, the best drying method is to blow dry with a brush and stand dryer but if the coat is trimmed, cabinet dryers can be used. All finishing, however, should be done with a stand dryer to ensure total removal of dead undercoat and tangles. Working to a routine on long coats is vitally important or you will become lost and miss areas. Use your free hand to hold the coat open. This allows you to brush the coat ensuring that it is dried straight. Always brush the area where the dryer is blowing.

WIRE COAT

Breed example: West Highland White (Te-Wi)

Most wire-coated breeds seen in a salon will not have correct textured coats due to clipping and/or poor coat quality. These dogs can be bathed with a regular shampoo and dried either in a cabinet dryer or using a stand dryer.

For correct textured coats, hand stripping must always be done prior to bathing. If you are hand stripping, it is not always necessary to bath the dog as the coat can be cleaned during the stripping process. If the coat is stripped down to the undercoat, the dog can be bathed, but if the topcoat remains it is advisable to use another cleansing method to stop the coat from lifting and appearing bushy.

To clean a wire coat, you can use dry shampoo powders or chalk but ensure that these are brushed thoroughly through the coat to prevent irritation. Spray-in coat conditioner can also be used with a good massage and a rubber brush to remove any dirt. You can shampoo the leg furnishings and beard to present a better-finished picture.

WOOL COAT

Breed example: Poodle (Ut-Wo)

Select an appropriate shampoo for the skin type. It is also good to use a conditioner with these coat types to assist in the specific blow drying techniques and to prevent breakage. Squeeze the excess water from the coat and use a blaster to remove the dead coat.

'Blow' or 'fluff' drying is a must for most wool-coated breeds to ensure the correct finish for the trimming techniques required. Always use the brush to deflect airflow (Fig. 9.1). Start drying at the head and ears 'ironing' out the curls with long brush strokes as you go. Continue down the body and the front legs and then the back legs and tail. The finished coat should be straight from the root outwards and stand out from the skin (Fig. 9.2).

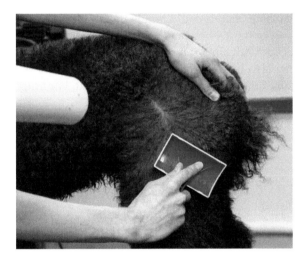

Fig. 9.1 Use a brush to deflect the airflow.

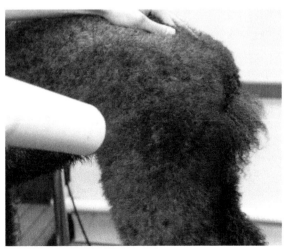

Fig. 9.2 The finished coat should be straight from the root.

Blow drying is a skilled technique that can take time to master so do not try to rush. If the coat is dry before you have been able to use the brush, spray the coat with water to enable you to achieve the correct finish.

SILK COAT

Breed example: Yorkshire Terrier (To-Si)

Shampoo the coat using a cleansing shampoo. Do not rub the coat as this could cause tangles. Follow the coat growth as you are shampooing to help penetration of the lather. After rinsing, apply a good quality conditioner; this will help the coat to fall and flow naturally and can help reduce static. If the coat is lacking condition, or is very knotty, allow the conditioner to soak in for five or ten minutes keeping the dog warm by wrapping it in a towel. Rinse thoroughly.

If the coat is long do not use the blaster as this could tangle the coat. However, do blast a shorter coat. For full long coats the best method of drying is to use a stand dryer to blow dry. Part the coat with clips if necessary to work systematically (Fig. 9.3). A cabinet dryer can also be used but the coat should always be finished with a stand dryer to ensure total dryness and a knot-free coat. For long coats there should be a centre parting down the back.

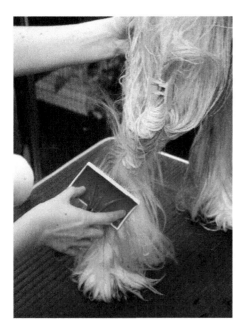

Fig. 9.3 Part the coat with clips if necessary.

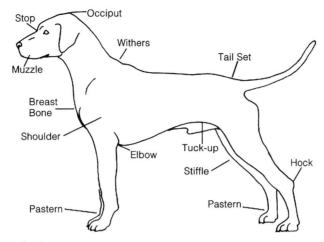

Fig. 9.4 Points of a dog.

GENERAL TERMINOLOGY

When trimming any dog it is useful to be aware of the basic anatomy (points) of a dog (Fig. 9.4). This will enable you to follow clipping/trimming lines and balance the trim, creating the best possible style and shape for the dog. It is not necessary to remember the name of every bone and muscle but the terms listed below will be of help.

Angulation	The angles formed by the bones meeting at a joint.
Balance	Most important. A symmetrical proportioned overall picture, i.e. balance of head to tail.
Beard	Long hair on the muzzle and under the jaw.
Blown	Refers to a moulting coat or a coat ready to hand strip.
Cat foot	Short, round, compact feet.
Cobby	Compact, short bodied.
Conformation	Structure of the dog.
Corkscrew tail	A twisted tail.
Cow hocks	Hock joints turned towards each other causing the feet to turn out.
Crest	Arched part of the neck.
Croup	Rump.
Expression	Appearance of the head and face.
Eyebrows	Hair above the eye.
Fall	Long hair around the head.
Feathering	Long hair on ears, legs and tail.
Flag	Long hair on tail.
Foreleg	From elbow to foot on the front legs.
Furnishings	Long hair on ears, legs and tail.
Gay tail	Tail carried high over the dog's back.

Guard hairs   Longer, stiffer hairs growing through the undercoat.
Hare foot   Two centre toes longer than the two outer toes.
Hind leg   Rear leg from the pelvis to the foot.
Hindquarter   Rear part of the dog.
Jowls   Fleshy parts of the lips and jaw.
Leather   Refers to the outer ear.
Loin   Area of body from the last rib to the hindquarter.
Low set   Tail set below the top line, ears set below the correct line for the breed.
Mane   Long hair on the side, top of the neck and chest.
Pads   Skin on the underside of the feet.
Profile   Side view of the dog.
Tail set   Position of the tail on the body.
Topknot   Woolly, silky or long hair on the top of the head.
Topline   Outline of the dog from the withers to the croup.
Withers   Highest point of the body at the top of the shoulder blades.

TRIMMING TIPS

When trimming, you should bear in mind that all dogs are different – even those of the same breed – and you should therefore consider the shape of the dog and work towards achieving the best possible look. Many faults on a dog can be disguised with clever trimming, e.g. cow hocks and bandy legs can be made to look straighter (Fig. 9.5).

While trimming you must remember to position yourself such that you can see the exact trimming line. Look straight at the line you are trimming and try to get the dog to stand four square to gain the best advantage and reduce chop marks and incorrect lines in the coat. When trimming the legs remember that there are four sides to trim (Fig. 9.6).

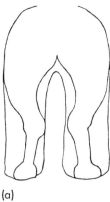
(a)

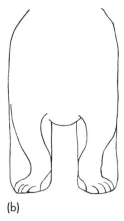
(b)

Fig. 9.5 (a) Cow hocks. (b) Bandy legs.

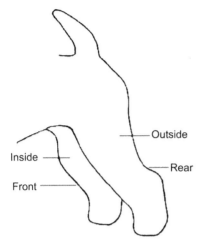

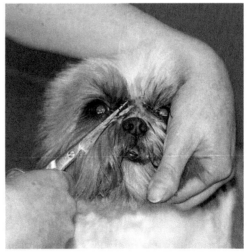

Fig. 9.6 Trimming legs – remember there are four sides to trim.

Trimming around the head on a fidgety dog can be difficult. Control the head by holding the beard or muzzle firmly (Fig. 9.7). **The safety of the dog is paramount**. Never point the scissors towards the eyes but always across them and be very aware of loose skin around this area (Fig. 9.8). When trimming around the ears always trim from the base towards the tip to ensure the ear is not cut with the heel of the scissors; use the tips of the scissors (Fig. 9.9). Keep your thumb close to the leather and work carefully around the edge (Fig. 9.10). Be very careful when using clippers around the ears. To avoid injury be aware of the danger areas indicated by red lines on Fig. 9.11.

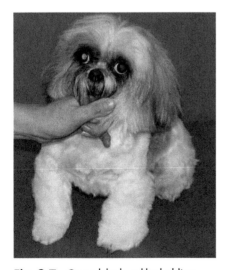

Fig. 9.7 Control the head by holding the muzzle.

Fig. 9.8 Always use scissors across the eye.

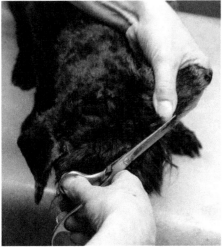

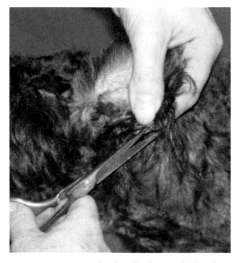

Fig. 9.9 Trimming around the ear.

Fig. 9.10 Keep the thumb close to the leather.

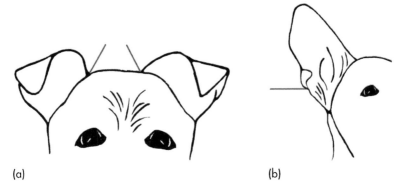

(a)

(b)

Fig. 9.11 Be aware of the danger areas while clipping.

Under the pads trimming can be done with either scissors or clippers. Whichever method is used, the finger hold shown in Fig. 9.12 will help to open the pad wide. Usually underpads can be trimmed with scissors but if the feet are matted, an ultra-fine blade (size 50) can be used to remove the mat (Fig. 9.13).

Great care should be taken when clipping around the groin and anal areas, as there could be a severe clipper reaction. Use a size 10 or 15 blade and clip carefully avoiding the nipples (Figs 9.14 and 9.15). **Never clip over the opening of the vulva or penis or directly over the anus**. Figs 9.16 and 9.17 illustrate how to correctly clip the area around the anus and groin.

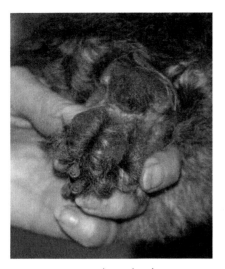

Fig. 9.12 Open the pad wide.

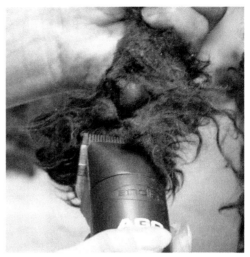

Fig. 9.13 Clippers used to remove the mat.

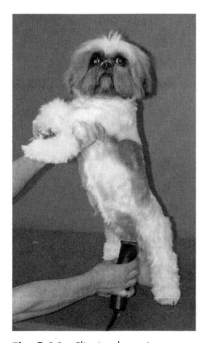

Fig. 9.14 Clipping the groin area.

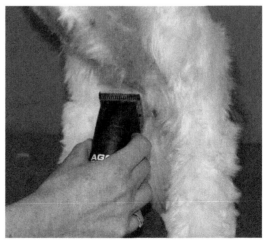

Fig. 9.15 Carefully avoid the nipples.

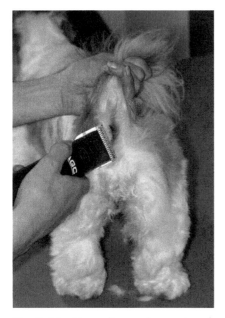 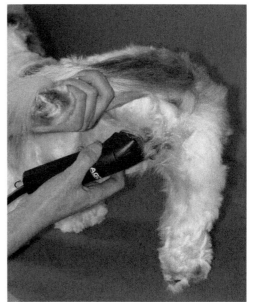

Fig. 9.16 Never clip over the opening of the anus.

Fig. 9.17 Never clip over the opening of the vulva.

SCISSORING FEET

Trim the nails first. The dog shown in Fig. 9.18a has very long nails. These should be clipped short before the feet are trimmed or shaped (Fig. 9.18b).

Round feet

Feet are trimmed in the way shown in Figs 9.19–9.22 when a dog has a full length coat, e.g. Bearded Collie (Pa-Dc2), Afghan Hound (Ho-Si), when the owner requires a neater edge. To achieve the required look, lift the leg coat out of the way and trim close to the front two toes (Fig. 9.19) and to the outer pads (Fig. 9.20) but NOT around the back of the foot. Stand the foot on the table and trim the overhang at the back of the foot (Fig. 9.21).

Tight feet

Tight feet are appropriate for West Highland White (Te-Wi) and Lhasa Apso (Ut-Dc2) in teddy bear trim and any other breeds with such trims. Lift the leg coat out of the way and trim tight around the front two toes (Fig. 9.23) and the outer pads (Fig. 9.24). Lift the leg and comb down the overhang at the back of the main pad and trim across (Fig. 9.25). The foot should blend into the leg trimming. Do not make the foot too small, as this will ruin the overall leg finish (Fig. 9.26).

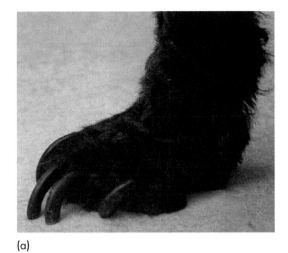

(a)

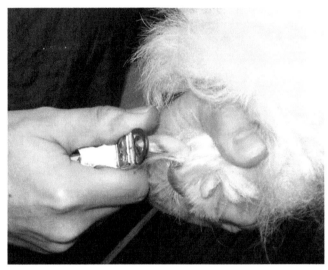

(b)

Fig. 9.18 (a) Over-long nails.
(b) Trimming the nails.

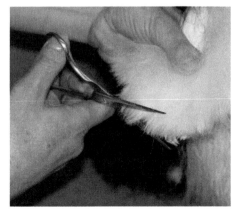

Fig. 9.19 Round foot trim: Step 1 – around the front two toes.

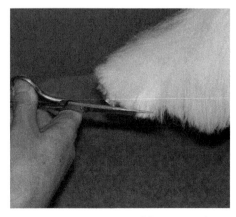

Fig. 9.20 Step 2 – around the outer pads.

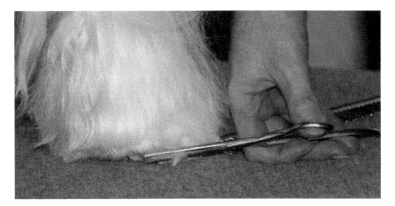

Fig. 9.21 Step 3 – around the back of the foot.

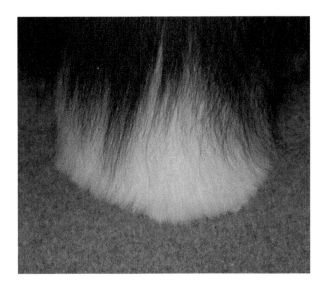

Fig. 9.22 Finished foot should look neat and tidy.

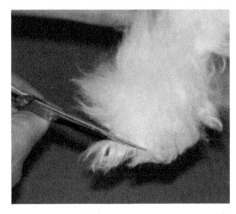

Fig. 9.23 Tight feet trim: Step 1 – trim round the front two toes.

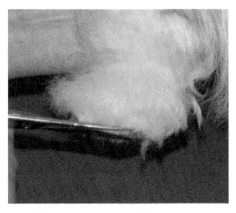

Fig. 9.24 Step 2 – around the outer pads.

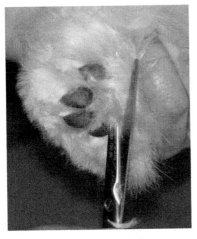

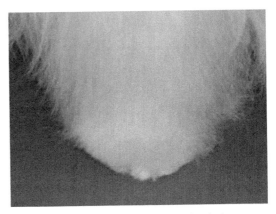

Fig. 9.25 Step 3 – comb down the overhang on the main pad and trim across.

Fig. 9.26 Finished foot should blend in the leg trimming.

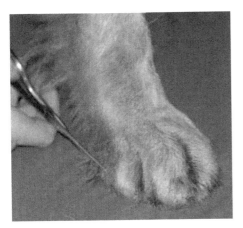

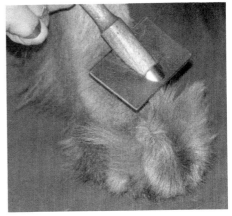

Fig. 9.27 Natural feet trim: Step 1 – trim outer edge of the foot.

Fig. 9.28 Step 2 – brush the hair up between the toes.

Natural feet

This look is appropriate for breeds such as Golden Retriever (Gd-Dc1), Border Collie (Pa-Dc1) and sometimes Cocker and Springer Spaniel (Gd-Si) depending on the length of the coat. To achieve this look, trim around the outer edge of the foot (Fig. 9.27), brush the hair upwards between the toes (Fig. 9.28) and trim or thin the excess coat level with the pastern hair (Fig. 9.29). Do not dig in the scissors or you will end up with chop marks. Tidy the overhang on the main pad (Fig. 9.30).

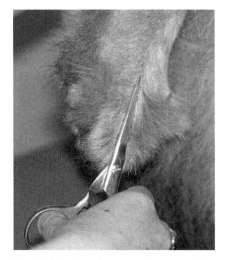

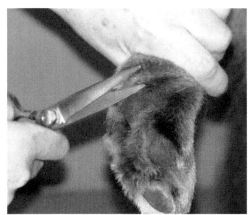

Fig. 9.29 Step 3 – cut or thin excess hair level with the pastern hair.

Fig. 9.30 Step 4 – tidy the overhang at the main pad.

Cat foot

The cat foot is mainly for spaniels. Start by trimming around the foot, keeping close to the front two toes (Fig. 9.31) and around the outer pads (Fig. 9.32). Use the hair on the top of the foot to build up padding on top of the toes (Fig. 9.33). Brush the hair upwards and cut or thin over the top but do not separate the pastern and foot hair (Fig. 9.34). Build the edge of the feet to a wall and trim the excess overhang hair from the main pad (Fig. 9.35). The finished foot is shown in Fig. 9.36.

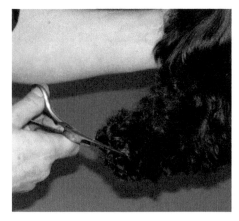

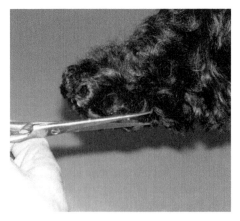

Fig. 9.31 Cat foot trim: Step 1 – start by trimming around the foot and keep close to the front two toes.

Fig. 9.32 Step 2 – around the outer pads.

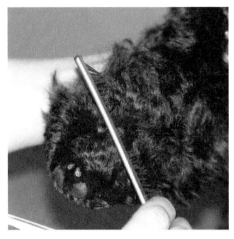

Fig. 9.33 Step 3 – use the hair on top of the toes.

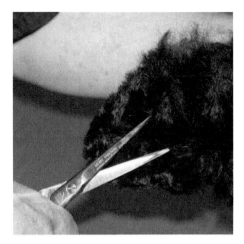

Fig. 9.34 Step 4 – do not separate the pastern and foot hair.

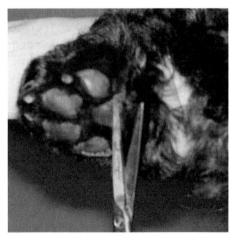

Fig. 9.35 Step 5 – build the edge of the feet to a wall and trim excess overhang from the main pad.

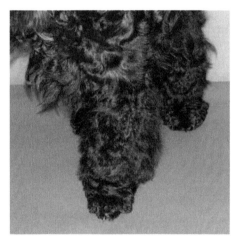

Fig. 9.36 Finished cat foot.

Padded hocks

The term 'padded hocks' is used in relation to some breeds. This term describes the area from the hock bone down to the main pad. To create a padded look, comb or brush the hair upwards and outwards and cut or thin the hair that extends beyond the hock bone (Fig. 9.37). This gives a solid shape to the leg rather than a spindly shape (Fig. 9.38).

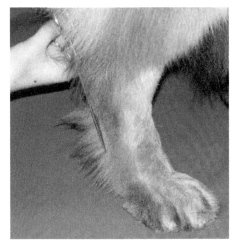

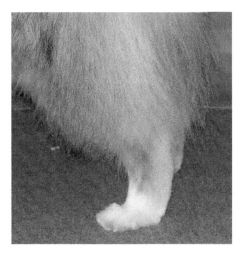

Fig. 9.37 Padded hocks: Comb or brush the hair upwards and cut or thin the hair.

Fig. 9.38 This gives a solid look to the leg.

LAYERING THE COAT

A coat is layered when you are trimming a long coat to a shorter length. It gives a very natural look to the dog and is appropriate for breeds such as Bearded Collie (Pa-Dc2), Lhasa Apso (Ut-Dc2) and Yorkshire Terrier (To-Si). To achieve the desired look, lift the coat with a comb and catch the hair between the fingers (Fig. 9.39), working in the direction of the coat growth. Use thinning scissors to trim the hair off – shorter towards the spine and longer towards the belly. Comb down to assess the finish.

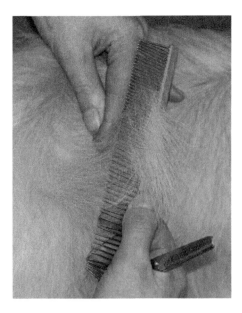

Fig. 9.39 Layer the coat by lifting the coat with a comb and catching between the fingers.

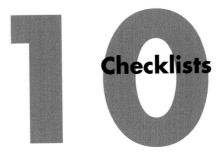

10 Checklists

HEALTH CHECKLIST

- Ears
- Teeth
- Skin and coat
- Anal glands
- Eyes
- Lumps and bumps
- Genital areas
- Weight loss or gain

PRE-TRIMMING CHECKLIST

- Health check
- Ensure total removal of knots and dead coat
- Bath and dry according to coat type
- Trim nails or claws
- Check ears

DOG BATHING CHECKLIST

Bath according to coat type. Have all your equipment to hand. Check the water temperature, prepare the shampoo and place the dog in the bath. For greater detail refer to Chapters 6 and 9.

Wet the dog thoroughly:

- Start behind the shoulders.
- Work backwards over the body, down the legs and tail.
- Finally wet the head.
- Work the water through the coat to ensure total saturation.
- Take care not to get water in the nose or ears (ear canal).

Check and empty the anal glands if necessary. Apply shampoo to:

- Tail.
- Back legs to the feet.
- Body and undercarriage.
- Front legs to feet.
- Shoulders and chest.
- Head and beard.

Then:

- Rinse the dog from head to tail.
- Second shampoo and second rinse.
- Conditioner if appropriate.
- Rinse thoroughly. Squeeze the excess water and towel dry the dog.

DOG DRYING CHECKLIST

For more details see Chapters 6 and 9.

- Use the method appropriate for the breed and coat type.
- Dry the coat thoroughly.
- Remove any knots or tangles.
- Remove dead undercoat.
- A final check through with comb.
- Keep your eyes open for lumps or bumps on the skin and skin rashes or differences in coat texture.

CAT BATHING CHECKLIST

For greater detail refer to Chapter 6.

- Have all your equipment to hand.
- Select an appropriate cat shampoo.
- Do not fasten a cat in the bath. Hold the cat by the scruff of the neck (let it rest its front feet on the edge of the bath if it wants to).
- Do NOT wet the cat's head.
- Shampoo starting from the neck, down the body to the tail, paying particular attention to the base of the tail.
- Shampoo the legs and remember to wash the feet.
- Wipe the head with a face cloth or small piece of absorbent cloth.
- Rinse thoroughly.
- Take four pieces of damp cotton wool and wipe around each ear and eye using one piece for each.
- Squeeze the excess water from the coat with a moisture absorbent cloth.
- Towel dry thoroughly.

CAT DRYING CHECKLIST

For more details see Chapter 6.

Cabinet drying

- Remove the cat after ten minutes, comb through and if the coat is still wet return to the cabinet for another ten minutes.
- A soft slicker brush can be used gently on the legs.
- Repeat the above until the cat is dry or finish as below.

Drying with a stand dryer

- Blow dry and comb or brush removing all tangles and dead coat.
- A soft slicker brush can be used gently on the legs.
- Remember that a cat's skin is much thinner and more sensitive than a dog's skin so do not be harsh.

HAND-STRIPPING CHECKLIST

- Health check.
- Strip coat prior to bathing.
- Bath if required.
- Complete hygiene clipping.
- Complete feet trimming.
- Complete nail check.
- Complete ear check.
- Minimal use of scissors or thinners to style of breed profile.

COLOUR CODING CHECKLIST

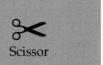

Scissor

Straight scissors
Thinning scissors
Foot scissors or any of a combination of these

Fine blade

Fine blades
Size range from 50 to 10
Or reverse 7F

Medium blade

Medium blade
Sizes range from 7F to 3F

Thinning and blending

Thinning and blending
Scissors or thinning scissors can be used

BLADE SIZES CHECKLIST

Blade number*

50 – Surgical, used for mainly show trims.
40 – As with '50'.
30 – Used for some thick-coated Terrier ears, Schnauzer ears and Poodle face and feet.
15 – Used for Poodle face, feet and tail.
10 – Hygiene clipping.
10 – West Highland White ear tips.
10 – Terrier and Spaniel head clipping.
9 – Short body clipping blades can be used for thick-coated Spaniel or long-legged Terrier bodies.
$8^{1}/_{2}$ – As with '9'.
7F – General Spaniel, Schnauzer, long-legged Terrier bodies.
5F – Poodle and West Highland White bodies.
4F – Longer general body clipping.
3F – As '4F'.

* The higher the number the shorter the blade cutting length.

TRIMMING CHECKLIST

- Complete fine clipping according to breed type.
- Hygiene clip (size no. 10 blade (not smooth coats)).
- Complete medium clipping or scissoring or thinning according to breed type.
- Trim legs, skirt, chest, head and tail. If clipping ears, use scissors around the edges to neaten.
- Check all work for balance and neatness.

CHECKLIST FOR MAINTENANCE OF EQUIPMENT

For greater detail refer to Chapter 2.

Clipper care

- Service – six months to one year.
- Do not wind flex around the clipper.
- Do not drop.
- Do not store in a damp environment.

Blade care

- Oil with a drop of oil or spray it.
- Disinfect regularly.
- Hold the clipper blade in a downward direction and spray working blades between the two plates.
- Wipe off excess oil.
- Never leave blades in the wash for more than a few minutes, wipe off any residue and dry.
- Check for broken teeth.
- Do not take blades apart.
- Equipment should be stored after cleaning and oiling or greasing.
- Sterilise each item after every dog.

Scissor care

- Scissors should never be shared.
- Clean scissors with fine machine oil such as clipper oil.
- Store each pair of scissors in a separate compartment.
- Scissors should never be dropped.
- Scissors should be serviced and sharpened by a competent professional.
- If you are left handed or have any hand/wrist problems tell the technician.

11 Breed Profiles

Afghan Hound (Ho-Si)
Airedale Terrier (Te-Wi)
American Cocker Spaniel (Gd-Si)

Bearded Collie (Pa-Dc2)
Bedlington Terrier (Te-Wo)
Bernese Mountain Dog (Wo-Dc1)
Bichon Frise (To-Wo)
Border Collie (Pa-Dc1 or Sm)
Border Terrier (Te-Wi)
Bouvier des Flandres (Wo-Dc2)
Boxer (Wo-Sm)

Cairn Terrier (Te-Wi)
Cavalier King Charles Spaniel (To-Si)
Chow Chow (Ut-Dc1)
Clumber Spaniel (Gd-Si)
Cocker Spaniel (Gd-Si)

Dachshund – Long Coat (Ho-Si)
Dachshund – Smooth Coat (Ho-Sm)
Dachshund – Wire Coat (Ho-Wi)
Dandie Dinmont Terrier (Te-Wi)
Deerhound (Ho-Wi)
Dobermann (Wo-Sm)

English Setter (Gd-Si)
English Springer (Gd-Si)

Field Spaniel (Gd-Si)
Flat Coat Retriever (Gd-Dc1)

German Shepherd (Pa-Dc1)
Giant Schnauzer (Wo-Wi)

Golden Retriever (Gd-Dc1)
Gordon Setter (Gd-Si)
Griffon Bruxellois (To-Wi or Sm)

Irish Setter (Gd-Si)
Irish Terrier (Te-Wi)
Irish Water Spaniel (Gd-Wo)
Irish Wolfhound (Ho-Wi)
Italian Spinone (Gd-Wi)

Kerry Blue Terrier (Te-Si)

Labrador Retriever (Gd-Dc1)
Lakeland Terrier (Te-Wi)
Lhasa Apso (Ut-Dc2)
Lowchen (To-Si)

Maltese (To-Si)
Miniature Schnauzer (Ut-Wi)

Newfoundland (Wo-Dc1)
Norfolk Terrier (Te-Wi)
Norwich Terrier (Te-Wi)

Old English Sheepdog (Pa-Dc2)

Papillion (To-Si)
Parson Russell Terrier (Te-Wi)
Pekingese (To-Dc1)
Polish Lowland Sheepdog (Pa-Dc2)
Pomeranian (To-Dc1)
Poodle (Ut-Wo)

Rough Collie (Pa-Dc1)

Samoyed (Pa-Dc1)
Schnauzer (Ut-Wi)

Scottish Terrier (Te-Wi)

Sealyham Terrier (Te-Wi)

Shetland Sheepdog (Pa-Dc1)

Shih Tzu (Ut-Dc2)

Soft Coated Wheaten Terrier (Te-Si)

St. Bernard (Wo-Dc1)

Sussex Spaniel (Gd-Si)

Tibetan Terrier (Ut-Dc2)

Welsh Springer Spaniel (Gd-Si)

Welsh Terrier (Te-Wi)

West Highland White Terrier (Te-Wi)

Wire Fox Terrier (Te-Wi)

Yorkshire Terrier (To-Si)

Crossbreeds

USE OF BREED PROFILES AND GROOMING TIPS

- Think about the dog you are trimming as an individual. Know about the characteristics of each breed as these differ from breed to breed, and the details will help you when styling and handling.
- **Two dogs of the same breed can vary enormously**.
- Use the trimming diagrams. Interpret them for the individual dog and think about making that dog look its best possible. There is no hard and fast rule for choosing the blade size – the size depends on the thickness of the dog's coat. Therefore gauge the coat's quality before you clip the body. Coats can be clipped with a skip-toothed blade which gives a longer finish than the 'F' blades, or they can be thinned or scissored to give a more natural or longer effect, respectively.
- When clipping, use the blending lines and the position of the tail set (see Fig. 9.4, Chapter 9) as the line to stop clipping. Then scissor or thin to give the desired finish for an overall and tidy blended trim.
- When trimming beards, lift the beard furnishings out of the way to tidy round the clipped area.
- When trimming eyebrows, lift the brow furnishings to clear in front of the eye corners.
- To give lift to long brows you can thin or scissor a little from the inner corner of the eyebrow furnishings.
- Never trim chest furnishings with the dog sitting down.
- When trimming ensure all clipping lines are precise and scissoring is even to give the dog the best possible look.
- Refer to Chapter 9 for points of the dog (Fig. 9.4) and terminology.
- Refer to Chapter 10 for working checklists.

Trims change over time so keep your knowledge of these changes up to date by attending seminars and dog shows.

THE BREEDS

The following breed appearance and characteristics have been reproduced by kind permission of the Kennel Club.

Afghan Hound (Ho-Si)

General appearance: Gives the impression of strength and dignity, combining speed and power. Head held proudly.

Characteristics: Eastern or oriental expression is typical of breed. The Afghan looks at and through one.

Recommended time between trims: 4–6 weeks.

Consult checklists in Chapter 10.

- The Afghan should look natural and untrimmed. Fig. 11.1 shows an Afghan before trimming. Compare this to the finished dog in Fig. 11.4.
- Scissor or clip under the pads.
- Strip any excess hair from the saddle (Fig. 11.2).

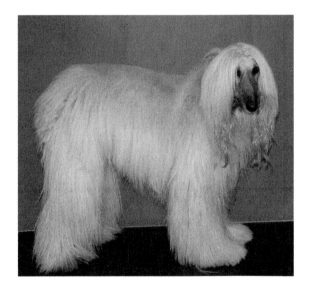

Fig. 11.1 Afghan before grooming.

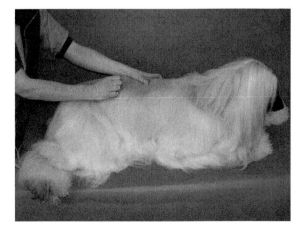

Fig. 11.2 Stripping the saddle.

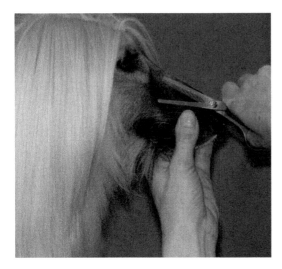

Fig. 11.3 Clearing the face.

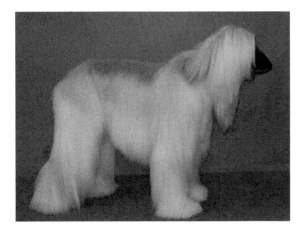

Fig. 11.4 Finished full-coated Afghan.

- Ensure that the face is smooth by stripping dead coat or using thinning scissors (Fig. 11.3).
- If requested, the feet can be trimmed into a round shape. Fig. 11.4 shows a finished Afghan.

Alternative method

Trimming this coat can be difficult as the texture of the coat shows scissor marks. If the legs are to be shortened, scissor down the coat following the natural flow of the coat growth and contours of the dog (Fig. 11.5). Thinning scissors can help reduce the 'chop marks' (Fig. 11.6). If the coat is badly matted, clipping may be the only option.

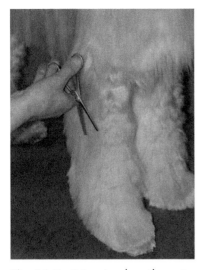

Fig. 11.5 Scissoring down the coat of an Afghan.

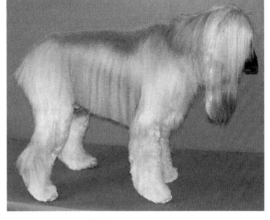

Fig. 11.6 Finished pet trim.

Airedale Terrier (Te-Wi)

General appearance: Largest of the Terriers, a muscular, active, fairly cobby dog, without suspicion of legginess or undue length of body.

Characteristics: Keen of expression, quick of movement, on the tiptoe of expectation at any moment. Character denoted and shown by expression of eyes and by carriage of ears and erect tail.

Recommended time between trims: 8–12 weeks.

Consult checklists in Chapter 10.

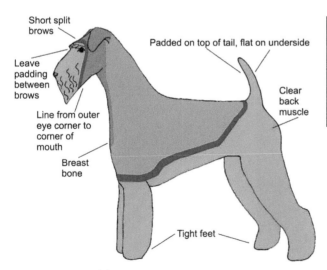

Short split brows

Leave padding between brows

Line from outer eye corner to corner of mouth

Breast bone

Padded on top of tail, flat on underside

Clear back muscle

Tight feet

Scissor or thinning scissors
Fine blade = 10 with the growth or 7F against the growth. Ears 15.
Medium blade = 7F
Blend with thinning scissors

Fig. 11.7 Airedale trim.

Hand stripping

The coat should be hand stripped all over to maintain the colour and texture. The process should never be uncomfortable for the dog, therefore stripping should be carried out when the coat is ready and should never be forced. You can assess the readiness of the coat by how it stands away from the body and by gently pulling a few hairs. If the coat is 'tight' to the body and the hair is difficult to pull out, it is not ready to strip.

Use either the finger and thumb or a stripping knife to remove the dead topcoat. Work to the pattern shown for clipping. The head, throat and ears need to be stripped very close so ensure you do not cause any friction with the knife. Clip inside the ears. Use thinning scissors to tidy the back muscle and around the feet. The head should be rectangular with short brows (Fig. 11.9).

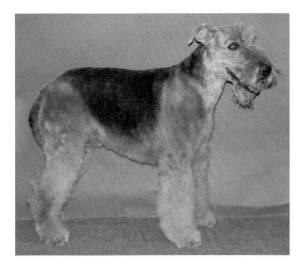

Fig. 11.8 Airedale Terrier: Pet trimmed.

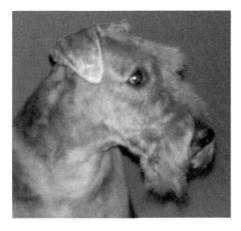

Fig. 11.9 Airedale Terrier: Trimmed head.

American Cocker Spaniel (Gd-Si)

General appearance: Serviceable-looking dog with refined chisel head, strong, well boned legs, well up at the shoulder, compact sturdy body, wide muscular quarters, well balanced.
Characteristics: Merry, free, sound, keen to work.
Recommended time between trims: 4–6 weeks.
Consult checklists in Chapter 10.

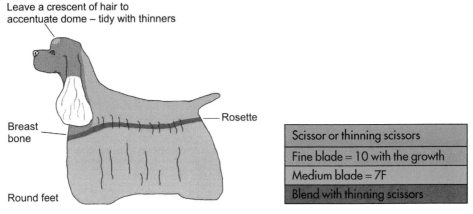

Fig. 11.10   American Cocker trim.

- The body coat should be hand stripped – strip dull, fluffy coat with finger and thumb.
- For pet trims the skirt can be taken down (made shorter) dramatically and the legs scissored to a tubular shape (Fig. 11.11).
- An undocked tail can be feathered or clipped very short.
- Fig. 11.12 is of an American Cocker Spaniel in show trim.

Bearded Collie (Pa-Dc2)

General appearance: Lean active dog, longer than it is high in approximate proportion of 5 to 4, measured from point of chest to point of buttock. Bitches may be slightly longer. Though strongly made, should show plenty of daylight under body and should not look too heavy. Bright enquiring expression is a distinctive feature.
Characteristics: Alert, lively, self-confident and active.
Recommended time between trims: 4–8 weeks.
Consult checklists in Chapter 10.

- A full-coated Bearded Collie should only have the hygiene areas and under the pads clipped.

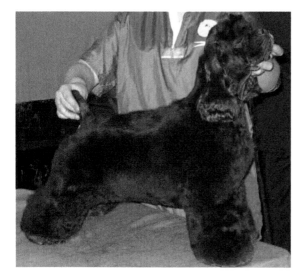

Fig. 11.11 American Cocker: Pet trimmed.

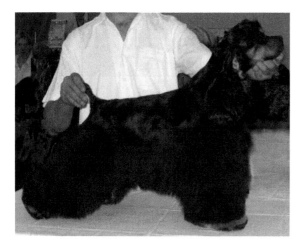

Fig. 11.12 American Cocker: Show trimmed.

- Most pet owners prefer the feet scissored round and a fringe cut into the topknot (Fig. 11.13). To trim the fringe, place your thumb on the stop and comb a small amount of coat forward and trim across from the outer corner of one eye to the outer corner of the other eye. Comb another section and trim the overhang.
- To take the coat down further you can layer the coat using thinning scissors. Lift one section of the coat at a time and layer, following the coat growth. Trim the edges of the legs to neaten and trim around the head shape.
- To shorten further clip the body coat (following the West Highland White body lines) and scissor the legs.
- If badly matted the coat may require complete clipping.

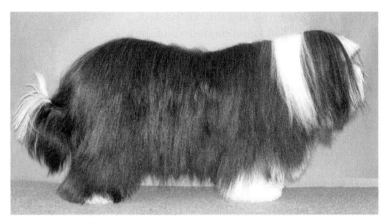

Fig. 11.13 Bearded Collie: Pet trimmed.

Bedlington Terrier (Te-Wo)

General appearance: A graceful, lithe, muscular dog, with no signs of either weakness or coarseness. Whole head pear- or wedge-shaped, and expression in repose mild and gentle.

Characteristics: Spirited and game, full of confidence. An intelligent companion with strong sporting instincts.

Recommended time between trims: 6–8 weeks.

Consult checklists in Chapter 10.

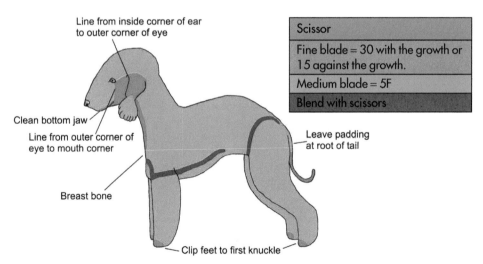

Fig. 11.14 Bedlington trim.

- The feet should be 'hare-like' and the tail 'rat-tail'.
- Scissor a diamond-shaped tassel on the end of the ear.

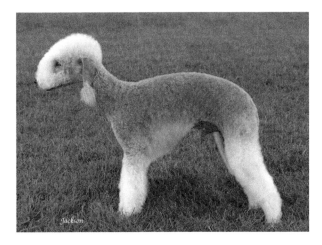

Fig. 11.15 Bedlington: Show presentation. (Photo courtesy of John D. Jackson.)

Bernese Mountain Dog (Wo-Dc1)

General appearance: Strong, sturdy working dog, active, alert, well-boned, of striking colour.
Characteristics: A multi-purpose farm dog capable of draught work. A kind and devoted family dog. Slow to mature.
Recommended time between trims: 3–4 months.
Consult checklists in Chapter 10.

- Trim natural feet with padded hocks.

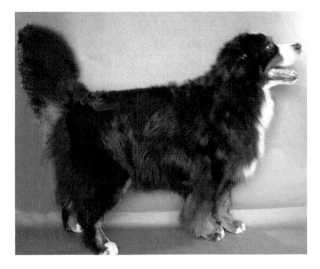

Fig. 11.16 Bernese: Pet tidy.

Bichon Frise (To-Wo)

General appearance: Well balanced dog of smart appearance, closely coated with handsome plume carried over the back. Natural white coat curling loosely. Head carriage proud and high.

Characteristics: Gay, happy, lively little dog.

Recommended time between trims: 4 weeks.

Consult checklists in Chapter 10.

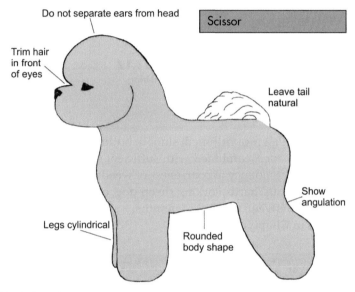

Do not separate ears from head

Scissor

Trim hair in front of eyes

Leave tail natural

Show angulation

Legs cylindrical

Rounded body shape

Fig. 11.17 Bichon trim.

• The coat should be ideally scissored to 7.5–10 cm (2–3 inches) in length. If a shorter trim is required you can clip the body with a 4F blade.

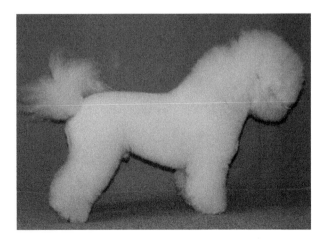

Fig. 11.18 Bichon: Full coated pet trim.

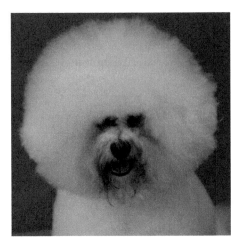

Fig. 11.19 Bichon: Full coated pet head trim.

Border Collie (Pa-Dc1 or Sm)

General appearance: Well proportioned, smooth outline showing quality, gracefulness and perfect balance, combined with sufficient substance to give impression of endurance. Any tendency to coarseness or weediness undesirable.
Characteristics: Tenacious, hard-working sheep-dog, of great tractability.
Recommended time between trims: 3–4 months.
Consult checklists in Chapter 10.

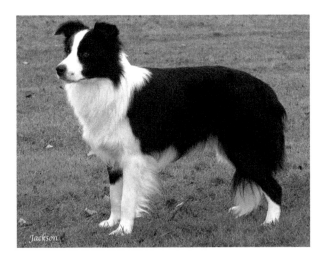

Fig. 11.20 Border Collie: Show or pet. (Photo courtesy of John D. Jackson.)

- Trim natural feet with padded hocks.
- Trim hair between the main pad and stopper pad.

Border Terrier (Te-Wi)

General appearance: Essentially a working terrier.
Characteristics: Capable of following a horse, combining activity with gameness.

Recommended time between trims: 3–4 months.
Consult checklists in Chapter 10.

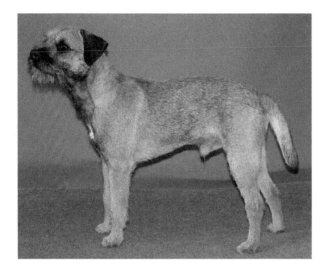

Fig. 11.21 Border Terrier:
Hand-stripped pet trim.

- Hand-strip the complete coat leaving small padded brows and rounded beard to create an 'otter head' appearance. However, if the skin is in poor condition or the coat is of poor texture hand-stripping may not always be appropriate as this could cause irritation.
- Clipping the coat is not advisable as this would cut into the undercoat and leave marks.
- Using thinning scissors all over the coat will create a more natural look.
- The beard and brow line should run from the outer corner of the eye to the corner of the mouth.
- If hand-stripping use thinning scissors to tidy under tail, around feet and rear muscle line.

Bouvier des Flandres (Wo-Dc2)

General appearance: Compact body, short coupled, powerfully built, well boned, strongly muscled limbs, giving impression of great power but without clumsiness in general deportment.
Characteristics: Lively appearance revealing intelligence, energy and audacity. Its harsh beard is very characteristic giving forbidding expression.
Recommended time between trims: 3–4 months.
Consult checklists in Chapter 10.

- Clip top of skull and ear with a fine blade size No. 10. Do *not* clip cheeks. Blend in beard with thinners.
- Use thinning scissors on the body and legs to shape to a natural conformation.
- Leave coat longer on the neck to create an arched neck.
- Trim throat shorter than body coat.

- Tidy under tail and back leg muscle.
- Tidy round feet.

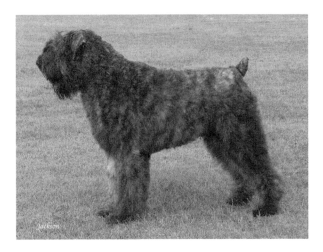

Fig. 11.22 Bouvier des Flandres: Show dog. (Photo courtesy of John D. Jackson.)

Boxer (Wo-Sm)

General appearance: Great nobility, smooth-coated, medium sized, square build, strong bone and evident, well-developed muscles.

Characteristics: Lively, strong, loyal to owner and family, but distrustful of strangers. Obedient, friendly at play, but with guarding instincts.

Recommended time between baths: 3–4 months.

Consult checklists in Chapter 10.

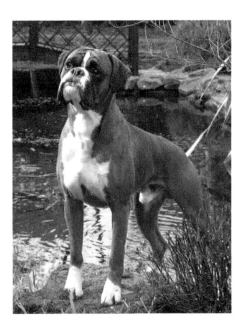

Fig. 11.23 Boxer: Show or pet. (Photo courtesy of John D. Jackson.)

Cairn Terrier (Te-Wi)

General appearance: Agile, alert, of workmanlike appearance. Standing well forward on forepaws. Strong quarters. Deep in rib, very free in movement. Weather-resistant coat.

Characteristics: Should impress as being active, game and hardy.

Recommended time between trims: 8–12 weeks.

Consult checklists in Chapter 10.

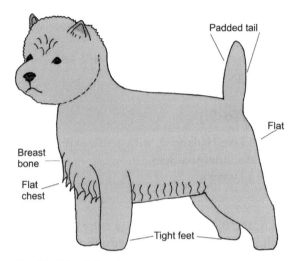

Padded tail

Flat

Breast bone

Flat chest

Tight feet

| Scissors and thinning scissors |
| Fine blade = 10. |

Fig. 11.24 Cairn trim.

- The entire coat should be hand-stripped.
- For pet purposes the use of thinners gives a much more natural appearance.

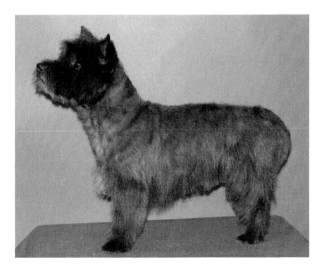

Fig. 11.25 Cairn: Pet trimmed.

Pet trim

- Follow a rounded head shape as shown for the West Highland White (Fig. 11.102 later). Trim the hair at the corner of the eye with thinning scissors, but do not over-trim here.
- Trim a fringe to create a visor over the eyes.
- The head should be a circular shape and all the hair should be of the same length.
- Scissor a semi-circle outline from the nose to behind the ear – the longest point being below the eye.
- Comb hair back and tidy any overhang at the back of the neck and ears with thinning scissors.
- Lift the hair on top of the head and sides in sections, using thinning scissors to create a circular shape (a layered full appearance).

Cavalier King Charles Spaniel (To-Si)

General appearance: Active, graceful and well balanced, with gentle expression.
Characteristics: Sporting, affectionate, absolutely fearless.
Recommended time between trims: 8–12 weeks.
Consult checklists in Chapter 10.

Do not clip this breed, in particular, the Blenheim and Ruby colorations. The undercoat is a different colour and clipper marks show very easily. Black and Tan and Tricolour do not look as bad but it is preferable that the body coat should be left natural. Use a Coat King or thinners to help the coat lay flat. If an owner insists on getting the body coat clipped, you do not have much choice!

- Trim natural feet.
- Tidy hock hair to look padded.
- Trim feathering to look natural and flowing.
- Thin all excessive coat under the ear to help with aeration.

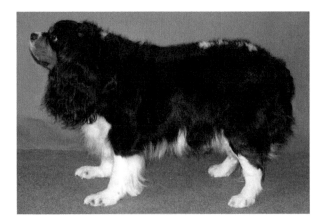

Fig. 11.26 Cavalier King Charles Spaniel: Pet trimmed.

Chow Chow (Ut-Dc1)

General appearance: Active, compact, short coupled and essentially well balanced, leonine in appearance, proud, dignified bearing; well knit frame; tail carried well over back.

Characteristics: Quiet dog, good guard, bluish-black tongue; unique in its stilted gate.

Recommended time between trims: 3–4 months.

Consult checklists in Chapter 10.

- Trim natural feet
- Trim padded hocks

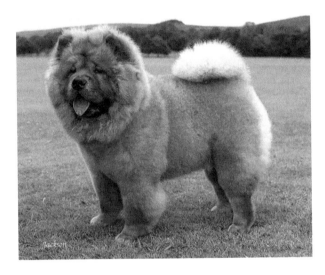

Fig. 11.27 Chow Chow: Show dog. (Photo courtesy of John D. Jackson.)

Clumber Spaniel (Gd-Si)

General appearance: Well balanced, heavily boned, active with a thoughtful expression, overall appearance denoting strength.

Characteristics: Stoical, great-hearted, highly intelligent with a determined attitude enhancing its natural ability. A silent worker with an excellent nose.

Recommended time between trims: 8–12 weeks.

Consult checklists in Chapter 10.

- Do not clip body coat. Hand-strip excessive coat or use Coat King or thinners to help coat look flat.
- Trim natural feet with padded hocks.
- Trim excess hair from ears and tidy edges.
- Trim feathering to look natural.
- Tidy throat area with thinning scissors.

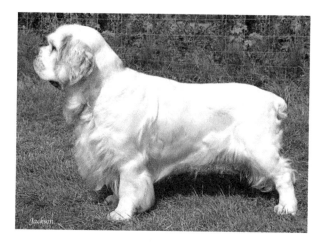

Fig. 11.28 Clumber Spaniel: Show dog. (Photo courtesy of John D. Jackson.)

Cocker Spaniel (Gd-Si)

General appearance: Merry, sturdy, sporting; well balanced; compact; measuring approximately same from withers to ground as from withers to root of tail.
Characteristics: Merry nature with ever-wagging tail, shows a typical bustling movement, particularly when following scent, fearless of heavy cover.
Recommended time between trims: 4–8 weeks.
Consult checklists in Chapter 10.

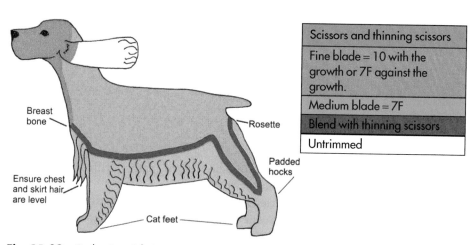

Fig. 11.29 Cocker Spaniel trim.

- When hand-stripping, remove dull and fluffy coat with finger and thumb.
- The coat should be hand-stripped but for pets clipping is very common.
- Trim cat feet with padded hocks.
- Feathering should look natural and flowing.
- An undocked tail should be trimmed to a flag shape.

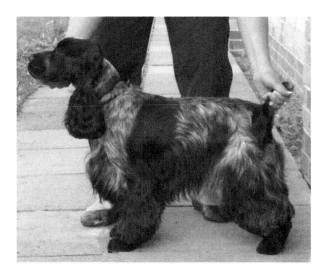

Fig. 11.30 Cocker Spaniel: Show trimmed pet.

Dachshund (Ho)

Long Coat (Si)

General appearance: Long and low, but with compact, well muscled body, bold, defiant carriage of head and intelligent expression.

Characteristics: Intelligent, lively, courageous to the point of rashness, obedient. Especially suited to going to ground because of low build, very strong fore quarters and fore legs. Long, strong jaw, and immense power of bite and hold. Excellent nose. Persevering hunter and tracker.

Recommended time between trims: 3–4 months.

Consult checklists in Chapter 10.

- Trim natural feet, padded hocks.
- If required thin out rear feathers and chest area using thinners or Coat King.

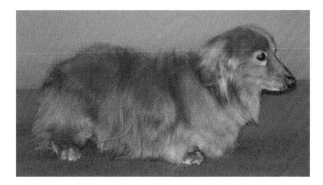

Fig. 11.31 Dachshund – Long Coat: Pet trimmed.

Smooth Coat (Sm)

General appearance: Long and low, but with compact, well muscled body, bold, defiant carriage of head and intelligent expression.
Characteristics: Intelligent, lively, courageous to the point of rashness, obedient. Especially suited to going to ground because of low build, very strong fore quarters and fore legs. Long, strong jaw, and immense power of bite and hold. Excellent nose. Persevering hunter and tracker.
Recommended time between baths: 4–6 months.
Consult checklists in Chapter 10.

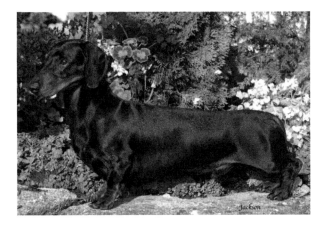

Fig. 11.32 Dachshund – Smooth Coat: Show dog. (Photo courtesy of John D. Jackson.)

Wire Coat (Wi)

General appearance: Long and low, but with compact, well muscled body, bold, defiant carriage of head and intelligent expression.
Characteristics: Intelligent, lively, courageous to the point of rashness, obedient. Especially suited to going to ground because of low build, very strong fore quarters and fore legs. Long, strong jaw, and immense power of bite and hold. Excellent nose. Persevering hunter and tracker.
Recommended time between trims: 4 months.
Consult checklists in Chapter 10.

- The coat should be completely stripped.
- You can assess the readiness of the coat by how it stands away from the body and by gently pulling a few hairs. If the coat is tight to the body and the hair is difficult to pull out, it is not ready to strip.
- If stripping is not possible, use thinning scissors to create a more natural look.
- Leave small padded brows and beard.

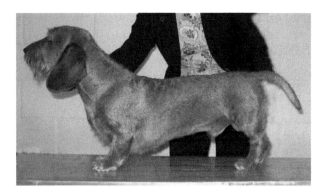

Fig. 11.33 Dachshund – Wire Coat: Hand-stripped pet trim.

Dandie Dinmont Terrier (Te-Wi)

General appearance: Distinctive head with beautiful silky covering, with large, wise, intelligent eyes offsetting long, low, weaselly body. Short, strong legs; weatherproof coat.
Characteristics: Game, workmanlike terrier.
Recommended time between trims: 3–4 months.
Consult checklists in Chapter 10.

- The entire coat should be hand-stripped.
- You can assess the readiness of the coat by how it stands away from the body and by gently pulling a few hairs. If the coat is tight to the body and the hair is difficult to pull out, it is not ready to strip.
- The front legs should be cylindrical in shape, flowing from the shoulder.
- The back legs need to be stripped clear at the back muscle.
- Trim tight feet.
- The tail should be flag-shaped.
- The skirt should be shaped tight to the groin and deep at the chest.
- The ears are stripped leaving a tassel at the end.

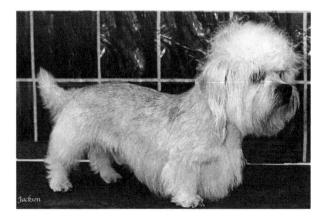

Fig. 11.34 Dandie Dinmont Terrier: Show dog. (Photo courtesy of John D. Jackson.)

- Clear the corners of the eyes and bridge of the nose with thinning scissors.
- Use thinning scissors to create a rounded head shape – trim under the ears to remove excessive coat and trim the beard so that it falls forwards.

Deerhound (Ho-Wi)

General appearance: Resembles a rough coated greyhound of larger size and bone.
Characteristics: The build suggests the unique combination of speed, power and endurance necessary to pull down a stag, but general bearing is one of gentle dignity.
Recommended time between trims: 6 months.
Consult checklists in Chapter 10.

- The coat should be hand-stripped to enhance the outline.
- Do not over-strip the coat. Just tidy all areas including the top of the head and the ears.
- Keep a rough-coated appearance.
- Use thinning scissors to trim tight feet.

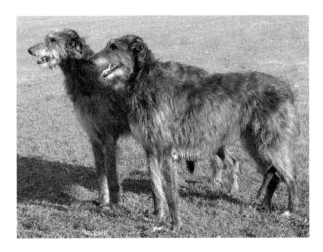

Fig. 11.35 Deerhound: Show dogs. (Photo courtesy of John D. Jackson.)

Dobermann (Wo-Sm)

General appearance: Medium size, muscular and elegant, with well set body. Of proud carriage, compact and tough. Capable of great speed.
Characteristics: Intelligent and firm of character, loyal and obedient.
Recommended time between baths: 3–4 months.
Consult checklists in Chapter 10.

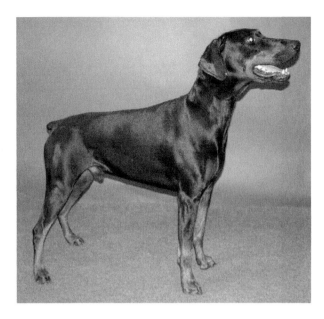

Fig. 11.36 Dobermann: Pet dog.

English Setter (Gd-Si)

General appearance: Of a medium height, clean in outline, elegant in appearance and movement. The Working English Setter may be proportionally lighter in build.

Characteristics: Very active with a keen game sense.

Recommended time between trims: 3–4 months.

Consult checklists in Chapter 10.

If the coat does not lay flat naturally, hand-strip, thin or use Coat King on the body coat. Do *not* clip the coat as this ruins the texture and appearance.

- Trim natural feet.
- Trim padded hocks.
- Tidy area between the main and stopper pads.
- Trim the tail so that it is flag-shaped.
- Strip, thin or clip the ears depending on the density of the coat. If clipping, use a 7F blade. Ensure you leave the front edge of the ear unclipped. Tidy this for a natural look to ensure a soft expression. Trim the ends and backs of the ears.
- Clip the throat area from the Adam's apple to the breast bone and blend along the seam line with thinners.

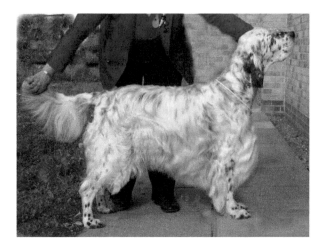

Fig. 11.37 English Setter: Hand-stripped pet dog in show trim.

English Springer (Gd-Si)

General appearance: Symmetrically built, compact, strong, merry, active. Highest on leg and raciest in build of all British land spaniels.

Characteristics: Breed is of ancient and pure origins, oldest of sporting gun dogs; original purpose was finding and springing game for net, falcon or greyhound. Now used to find, flush and retrieve game for gun.

Recommended time between trims: 8–12 weeks.

Consult checklists in Chapter 10.

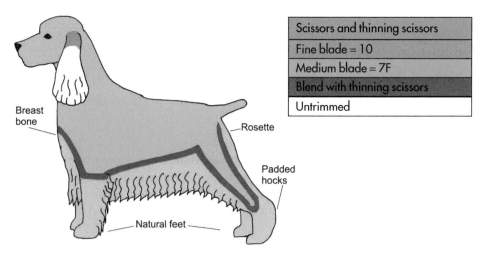

Scissors and thinning scissors
Fine blade = 10
Medium blade = 7F
Blend with thinning scissors
Untrimmed

Fig. 11.38 English Springer trim.

- This coat should be hand-stripped unless the dog is neutered (see below). Remove dull, fluffy coat with finger and thumb. If the coat lies flat naturally do not clip unless requested by the owner.
- A neutered dog may have a very fluffy, pale-coloured coat. Clipping is often the only option for these dogs as hand-stripping will not be successful.
- Trim natural feet.
- Trim padded hocks.
- An undocked tail should be trimmed so that it is flag-shaped.
- The overall effect should be natural and flowing (Fig. 11.39).
- Many owners prefer a much closer, shorter trim. This can include clipping ears and scissoring all feathers very short (Fig. 11.40).

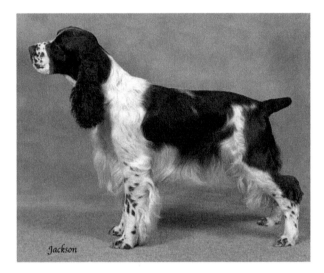

Fig. 11.39 English Springer: Show dog. (Photo courtesy of John D. Jackson.)

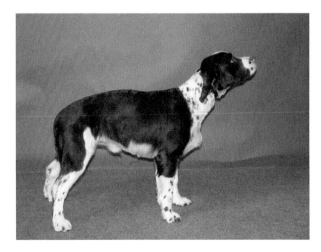

Fig. 11.40 English Springer: Very short pet trim.

Field Spaniel (Gd-Si)

General appearance: Well balanced, noble, understanding sporting spaniel built for activity and endurance.
Characteristics: Ideal for rough shooting or champion for the country dweller. Not suitable for city.
Recommended time between trims: 8–12 weeks.
Consult checklists in Chapter 10.

- For trimming guidelines see the Springer Spaniel colour sketch (Fig. 11.38).
- This coat should be hand-stripped unless the dog has been neutered (see below). Remove dull, fluffy coat with finger and thumb. If the coat lays flat naturally do not clip unless requested by the owner.
- A neutered dog may have a very fluffy, pale coloured coat. Clipping is often the only option for these dogs as hand-stripping will not be successful.
- Trim natural feet.
- Trim hocks tight.
- An undocked tail should be trimmed so that it is flag-shaped.
- The overall effect should be natural and flowing.

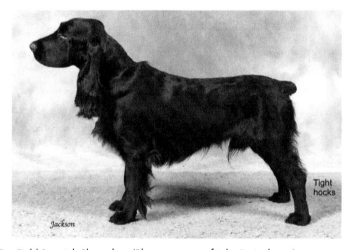

Fig. 11.41 Field Spaniel: Show dog. (Photo courtesy of John D. Jackson.)

Flat Coated Retriever (Gd-Dc1)

General appearance: A bright, active dog of medium size with an intelligent expression, showing power without lumber, and raciness without weediness.
Characteristics: Generously endowed with natural gun dog ability, optimism and friendliness demonstrated by enthusiastic tail action.
Recommended time between trims: 3–4 months.
Consult checklists in Chapter 10.

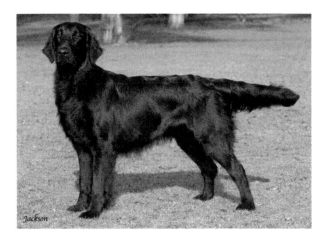

Fig. 11.42 Flat Coated Retriever: Show dog. (Photo courtesy of John D. Jackson.)

- Trim natural feet.
- Trim padded hocks.
- Strip or thin excessive hair on ears.

German Shepherd (Pa-Dc1)

General appearance: Slightly long in comparison to height; of powerful, well-muscled build with weather-resistant coat. Relationship between height, length, position and structure of fore- and hind quarters (angulation) producing far-reaching, enduring gait. Clear definition of masculinity and femininity essential, and working ability never sacrificed for mere beauty.

Characteristics: Versatile working dog, balanced and free from exaggeration. Attentive, alert, resilient and tireless with keen scenting ability.

Recommended time between trims: 3–4 months.

Consult checklists in Chapter 10.

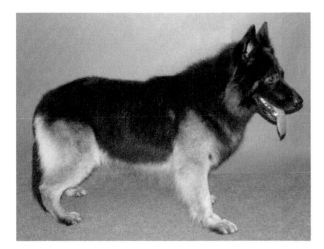

Fig. 11.43 German Shepherd: Pet dog.

- Long coated – trim natural feet and padded hocks.
- Use Coat King or thinners on the rear feathering if required.

Giant Schnauzer (Wo-Wi)

General appearance: Powerfully built, robust, sinewy, appearing almost square. Imposing, with keen expression and alert attitude. Correct conformation of the utmost importance.

Characteristics: Versatile, strong, hardy, intelligent and vigorous. Adaptable, capable of great speed and endurance and resistant to weather.

Recommended time between trims: 3 months.

Consult checklists in Chapter 10.

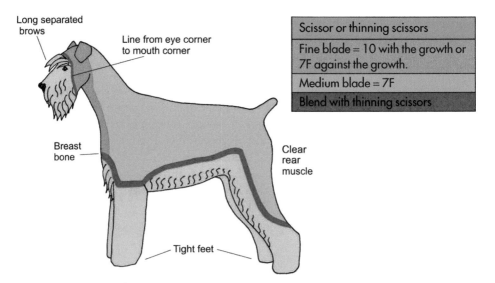

Fig. 11.44 Giant Schnauzer trim.

- The body coat should be hand-stripped.
- You can assess the readiness of the coat by how it stands away from the body and by gently pulling a few hairs. If the coat is tight to the body and the hair is difficult to pull out, it is not ready to strip.
- Clip the head, throat and chest even on a hand-stripped coat.
- Trim tight feet.
- Ensure rear muscle line perfectly free from hair.

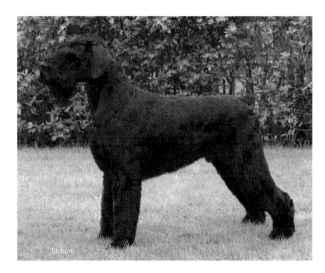

Fig. 11.45 Giant Schnauzer: Show dog. (Photo courtesy of John D. Jackson.)

Golden Retriever (Gd-Dc1)

General appearance: Symmetrical, balanced, active, powerful, level mover; sound with kindly expression.

Characteristics: Biddable, intelligent and possessing natural working ability.

Recommended time between trims: 3 months.

Consult checklists in Chapter 10.

- Trim natural feet.
- Trim padded hocks.
- Trim tail to flag shape.
- Tidy between main and stopper pads.
- Thin excessive coat around throat.
- Thin excessive feathering on ears. Ensure front of ear is left natural to keep a soft expression.

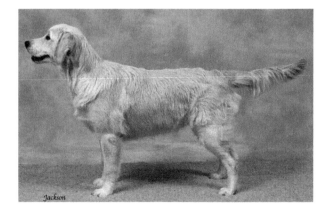

Fig. 11.46 Golden Retriever: Show dog. (Photo courtesy of John D. Jackson.)

Gordon Setter (Gd-Si)

General appearance: Stylish dog, with galloping lines. Consistent with its build which can be compared to a weight-carrying hunter. Symmetrical in confirmation throughout.
Characteristics: Intelligent, able and dignified.
Recommended time between trims: 3 months.
Consult checklists in Chapter 10.

- Trim natural feet.
- Thin excess hair from throat.

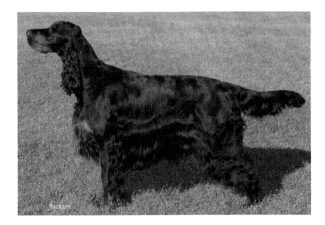

Fig. 11.47 Gordon Setter: Show dog.

Griffon Bruxellois (To-Wi or Sm)

General appearance: A cobby, well-balanced, square little dog, giving appearance of measuring the same from withers to tail root as from withers to ground.
Characteristics: Smart little dog with disposition of a terrier. Two varieties, rough coated, Griffon Bruxellois, and the smooth coated, Petit Brabancon. Both with pert, monkey-like expression, heavy for size.

Rough coated

Recommended time between trims: 3 months.
Consult checklists in Chapter 10.

- The coat should be hand-stripped all over. However, if the skin is in poor condition or the coat is of poor texture hand-stripping may not always be appropriate as this could cause irritation.
- You can assess the readiness of the coat by how it stands away from the body and by gently pulling a few hairs. If the coat is tight to the body and the hair is difficult to pull out, it is not ready to strip.

- Leave a light padding on legs.
- Tight feet.
- Use thinning scissors to tidy rear muscle line.
- Hand-strip the head and ears clean, leaving a full face and beard.

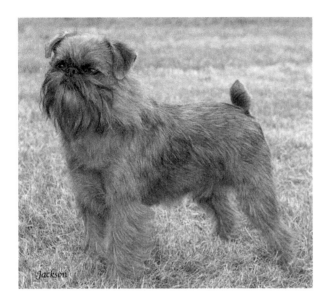

Fig. 11.48   Griffon Bruxellois – rough coat: Show dog. (Photo courtesy of John D. Jackson.)

Smooth coated

Recommended time between baths: 3–4 months.
Consult checklists in Chapter 10.

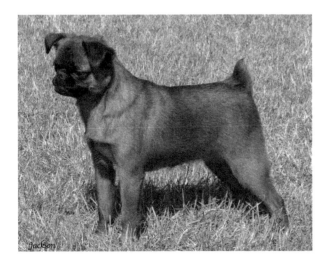

Fig. 11.49   Griffon Bruxellois – smooth coat: Show dog. (Photo courtesy of John D. Jackson.)

Irish Setter (Gd-Si)

General appearance: Must be racy, balanced and full of quality. In conformation, proportionate.

Characteristics: Most handsome, and refined in looks, tremendously active with untiring readiness to range and hunt under any conditions.

Recommended time between trims: 3 months.

Consult checklists in Chapter 10.

- The coat must not be normally clipped as this ruins the texture and appearance. Clipping should only be done as a last resort if the owner requests it.
- If the coat does not lay flat naturally, hand-strip or use Coat King to remove straggly ends.
- If the dog is neutered the coat may become dull and lifeless. Try using a Coat King or stripping knife to remove the dead looking coat.
- Trim natural feet.
- Trim padded hocks.
- Tidy area between the main and stopper pads.
- Trim tail to flag shape.
- Strip, thin or clip the ears depending on the density of the coat. If clipping, use a 7F blade. Ensure you leave the front edge of the ear unclipped – tidy this to a natural look to ensure a soft expression. Trim the end and back of the ear.
- Clip the throat area from the Adam's apple to the breast bone and blend along the seam line with thinners.

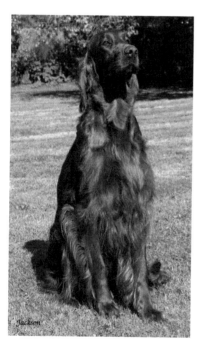

Fig. 11.50 Irish Setter: Show dog. (Photo courtesy of John D. Jackson.)

Irish Terrier (Te-Wi)

General appearance: An active, lively and wiry appearance; plenty of substance but free of clumsiness. Neither cloddy or cobby but showing a graceful racy outline.

Characteristics: There is a heedless, reckless pluck about the Irish Terrier which is characteristic and, coupled with the headlong dash, blind to all consequences, with which he rushes at his adversary, has earned for the breed the proud epitaph of 'the Daredevils'. When 'off duty' they are characterised by a quiet caress-inviting appearance, and when one sees them endearingly, timidly pushing their heads into their masters' hands, it is difficult to realise that on occasions, at the 'set-on', they prove that they have the courage of a lion, and will fight to the last breath in their bodies. They develop an extraordinary devotion for, and have been known to track their masters for almost incredible distances.

Recommended time between trims: 3 months.

Consult checklists in Chapter 10.

- The coat should be completely hand-stripped. However, if the coat is not suitable for hand-stripping due to poor skin condition or poor coat texture, use thinning scissors to create a more natural look.
- Clipping the coat is not advisable as this will cut into the undercoat and leave unsightly clipper marks.
- You can assess the readiness of the coat by how it stands away from the body and by gently pulling a few hairs. If the coat is tight to the body and the hair is difficult to pull out, it is not ready to strip.
- Clear muscle on rear leg and leave padded coat on bottom of leg and stifle.
- A short skirt can be left.
- Leave padded front legs.
- The head should have short, separated padded brows and a slight beard.

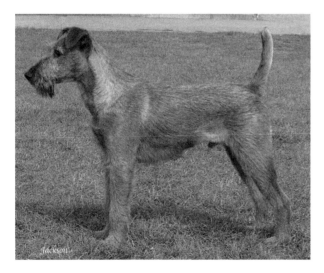

Fig. 11.51   Irish Terrier: Show dog. (Photo courtesy of John D. Jackson.)

Irish Water Spaniel (Gd-Wo)

General appearance: Smart, understanding, strongly built, compact.
Characteristics: Enduring, versatile gundog for all types of shooting, particularly in wildfowling.
Recommended time between trims: 6–8 weeks.
Consult checklists in Chapter 10.

- Dry the coat to maintain the natural wave.
- Clip the excessive coat on the tail with a no. 10 blade leaving the hair at the base.
- Clip the neck with a 7F blade against the growth up to the Adam's Apple – leave the beard under the jaw.
- Scissor the entire coat to follow and accentuate the dog's natural outline. Leave longer hair on the neck.
- Blend the topknot across the ears and leave a fringe over the eyes.

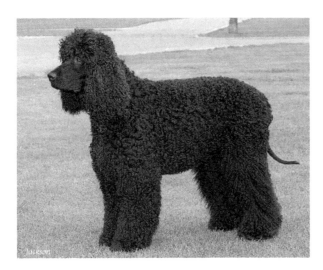

Fig. 11.52 Irish Water Spaniel: Show dog. (Photo courtesy of John D. Jackson.)

Irish Wolfhound (Ho-Wi)

General appearance: Of great size, strength, symmetry and commanding appearance, very muscular, yet gracefully built.
Characteristics: Of great power, activity, speed and courage.
Recommended time between trims: 6 months.
Consult checklists in Chapter 10.

- The coat should be hand-stripped to enhance the outline. Do not over-strip the coat. Just tidy all areas including top of head and ears. Keep a rough-coated appearance.

- You can assess the readiness of the coat by how it stands away from the body and by gently pulling a few hairs. If the coat is tight to the body and the hair is difficult to pull out, it is not ready to strip.
- Use thinning scissors to trim tight feet.

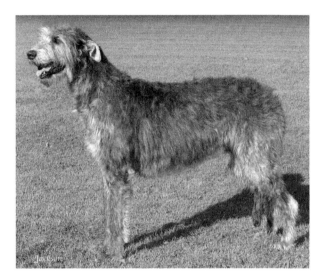

Fig. 11.53 Irish Wolfhound: Show dog. (Photo courtesy of John D. Jackson.)

Italian Spinone (Gd-Wi)

General appearance: Solid, squarely built, strong bone and well muscled. Kind and earnest expression.
Characteristics: Intrepid and untiring, very hardy, adaptable to any terrain including water. All-purpose gundog.
Recommended time between trims: 3–4 months.
Consult checklists in Chapter 10.

- The entire coat should be hand-stripped.
- You can assess the readiness of the coat by how it stands away from the body and by gently pulling a few hairs. If the coat is tight to the body and the hair is difficult to pull out, it is not ready to strip.
- Leave padded leg furnishings but thin out the coat from the middle of the thigh.
- Tidy round the feet and hock area to neaten.
- Ensure the tail remains thick.
- Hand-strip the head leaving the eyebrows and beard. The eyebrows should fan out and not be too pronounced. The foreface should be full.
- Leave a little feathering at the bottom of the ear.
- Ensure that the throat is clear from excessive coat.

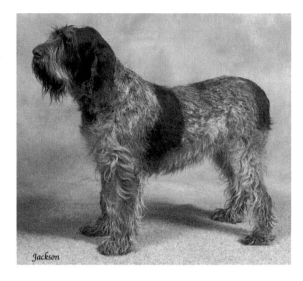

Fig. 11.54 Italian Spinone: Show dog. (Photo courtesy of John D. Jackson.)

Kerry Blue Terrier (Te-Si)

General appearance: Upstanding, well knit and proportioned, well developed and muscular body.

Characteristics: Compact, powerful Terrier, showing gracefulness and an aptitude of alert determination, with definite terrier style and character throughout.

Recommended time between trims: 4–6 weeks.

Consult checklists in Chapter 10.

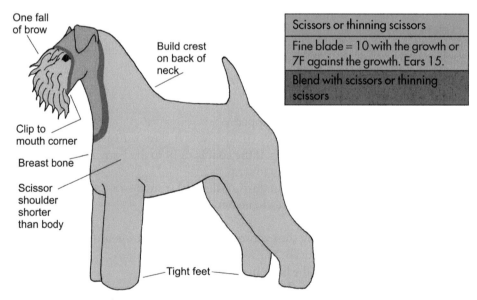

One fall of brow

Build crest on back of neck

Clip to mouth corner

Breast bone

Scissor shoulder shorter than body

Tight feet

Scissors or thinning scissors

Fine blade = 10 with the growth or 7F against the growth. Ears 15.

Blend with scissors or thinning scissors

Fig. 11.55 Kerry Blue trim.

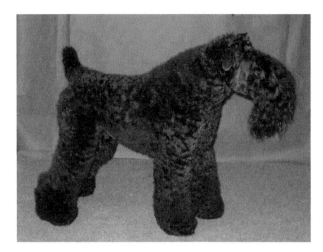

Fig. 11.56 Kerry Blue Terrier: Scissored pet trim.

- Dry the coat to maintain the natural wave.
- For pet trim, the body coat could be clipped with a no. 5F blade.

Labrador Retriever (Gd-Dc1)

General appearance: Strongly built, short coupled, very active; broad in skull; broad and deep through chest and ribs; broad and strong over loin and hind quarters.

Characteristics: Good tempered, very agile. Excellent nose, soft mouth; keen love of water. Adaptable, devoted companion.

Recommended time between baths: 3–4 months.

Consult checklists in Chapter 10.

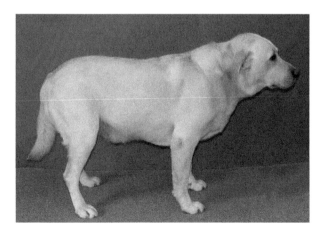

Fig. 11.57 Labrador Retriever: Pet dog.

Lakeland Terrier (Te-Wi)

General appearance: Smart, workmanlike, well balanced and compact.
Characteristics: Gay, fearless demeanour, keen of expression, quick of movement, on the tiptoe of expectation.
Recommended time between trims: 8–12 weeks.
Consult checklists in Chapter 10.

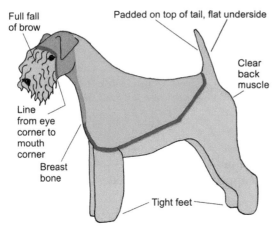

Scissors or thinning scissors
Fine blade = 10 with the growth or 7F against the growth. Ears 15.
Medium blade = 7F
Blend with thinning scissors

Fig. 11.58 Lakeland Terrier trim.

- The entire coat should be hand-stripped.
- You can assess the readiness of the coat by how it stands away from the body and by gently pulling a few hairs. If the coat is tight to the body and the hair is difficult to pull out, it is not ready to strip.
- Scissor or thinning scissor at the outer edge of the eye.

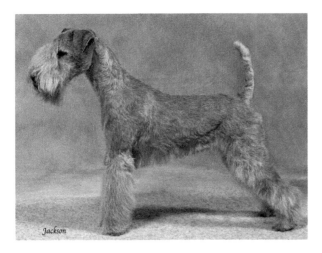

Fig. 11.59 Lakeland Terrier: Show dog. (Photo courtesy of John D. Jackson.)

Lhasa Apso (Ut-Dc2)

General appearance: Well balanced, sturdy, heavily coated.
Characteristics: Gay and assertive.
Recommended time between trims: 4–8 weeks.
Consult checklists in Chapter 10.

- A full-coated Lhasa Apso should only have the hygiene areas and under the pads clipped.
- If badly matted the coat may require complete clipping.
- Most pet owners prefer the feet scissored round and a fringe cut into the topknot (Fig. 11.60). To trim the fringe, place your thumb onto the stop and comb a small amount of coat forward and trim across from the outer corner of one eye to the outer corner of the other eye. Comb another section and trim the overhang.
- To take the coat down further you can layer the coat using thinning scissors. Lift one section of the coat at a time and layer, following the coat growth. Trim the edges of the legs to neaten and trim around the head shape.
- To shorten further clip the body coat (following the West Highland White body lines) and scissor the legs (Fig. 11.61).

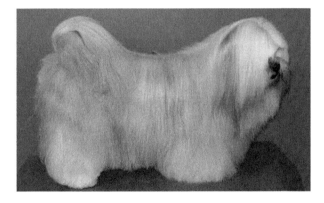

Fig. 11.60 Lhaso Apso: Pet dog in full coat.

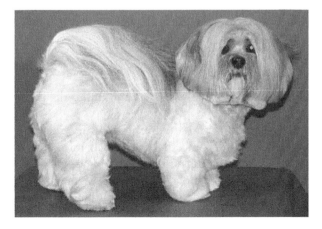

Fig. 11.61 Lhaso Apso: Teddy bear pet trim.

Lowchen (To-Si)

General appearance: Coat clipped in traditional lion clip, tail also clipped, topped with plume, giving appearance of a little lion. Strongly built, active, well balanced and alert.
Characteristics: Gay, happy, lively little dog.
Recommended time between trims: 4–8 weeks.
Consult checklists in Chapter 10.

- Should traditionally be in a lion clip, however most pet owners prefer either a full length of coat or a teddy bear trim (Fig. 11.62).
- To take the coat down further you can layer the coat using thinning scissors. Lift one section of the coat at a time and layer, following the coat growth. Trim the edges of the legs to neaten and trim around the head shape.
- To shorten further clip the body coat (following the West Highland White body lines) and scissor the legs.
- If badly matted the coat may require complete clipping.

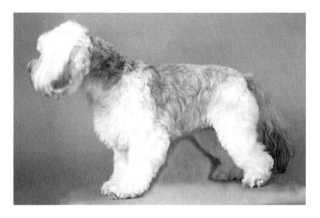

Fig. 11.62 Lowchen: Pet trimmed dog.

Maltese (To-Si)

General appearance: Smart, white coated dog, with proud head carriage.
Characteristics: Lively, intelligent, alert.
Recommended time between baths: 4–8 weeks.
Consult checklists in Chapter 10.

- A full-coated Maltese should only have the hygiene areas and under the pads clipped (Fig. 11.63).
- Most pet owners prefer the feet scissored round and a fringe cut into the top-knot. To trim the fringe, place your thumb onto the stop and comb a small amount of coat forward and trim across from the outer corner of one eye to the outer corner of the other eye. Comb another section and trim the overhang.
- To take the coat down further you can layer the coat using thinning scissors. Lift one section of the coat at a time and layer, following the coat growth. Trim the edges of the legs to neaten and trim around the head shape.

- To shorten further clip the body coat (following the West Highland White body lines) and scissor the legs.
- If badly matted the coat may require complete clipping.

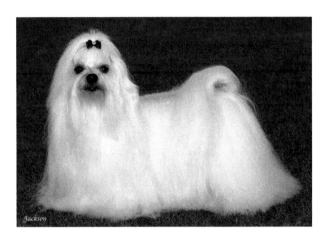

Fig. 11.63 Maltese: Show dog. (Photo courtesy of John D. Jackson.)

Miniature Schnauzer (Ut-Wi)

General appearance: Sturdily built, robust, sinewy, nearly square (length of body equal to height at shoulder). Expression keen and attitude alert. Correct conformation is of more importance than colour or other purely 'beauty' points.
Characteristics: Well balanced, smart, stylish and adaptable.
Recommended time between trims: 6–12 weeks.
Consult checklists in Chapter 10.

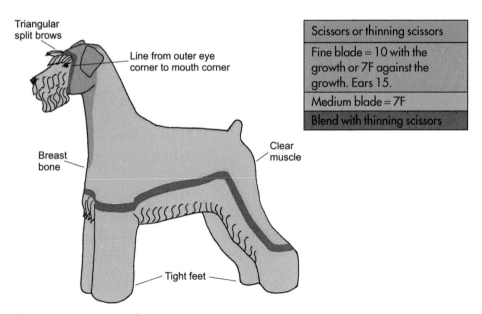

Fig. 11.64 Miniature Schnauzer trim.

- The coat should be hand-stripped. However, the head, throat and rear leg muscle should be clipped.
- Undocked tails should be clipped short.

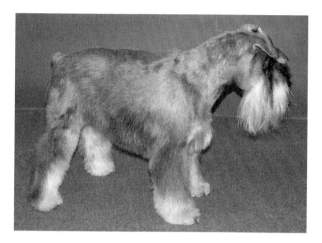

Fig. 11.65 Miniature Schnauzer: Clipped pet trim.

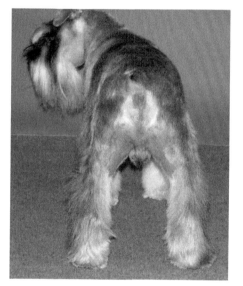

Fig. 11.66 Miniature Schnauzer: Shows clear back muscle.

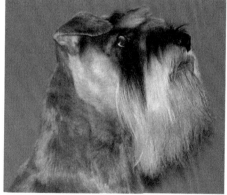

Fig. 11.67 Miniature Schnauzer: Pet trimmed head.

Newfoundland (Wo-Dc1)

General appearance: Well balanced, impresses with strength and great activity. Massive bone throughout, but not giving heavy inactive appearance. Noble, majestic and powerful.

Characteristics: Large draught and water dog, with natural life-saving instinct and devoted companion.

Recommended time between trims: 3–4 months.
Consult checklists in Chapter 10.

- Tidy natural feet.
- Tidy hocks.
- Then trim rear feathering and chest with thinners or Coat King if required.
- Strip or thin excessive hair around ears.

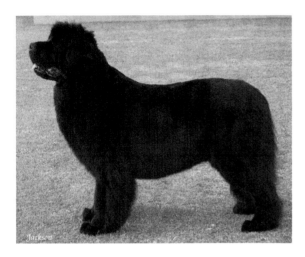

Fig. 11.68 Newfoundland: Show dog. (Photo courtesy of John D. Jackson.)

Norfolk Terrier (Te-Wi)

General appearance: Small, low, keen dog, compact and strong, short back, good substance and bone. Honourable scars from fair wear and tear permissible.
Characteristics: One of the smallest of terriers, a 'demon' for its size. Loveable disposition, not quarrelsome, hardy constitution.
Recommended time between trims: 3–4 months.
Consult checklists in Chapter 10.

- The entire coat should be hand-stripped. However, if the skin is in poor condition or the coat is of poor texture hand-stripping may not always be appropriate as this could cause irritation.
- Using thinning scissors all over the coat will create a more natural look.
- Clipping the coat is not advisable as this would cut into the undercoat and leave marks.
- You can assess the readiness of the coat by how it stands away from the body and by gently pulling a few hairs. If the coat is tight to the body and the hair is difficult to pull out, it is not ready to strip.
- Leave a little feathering on the rear and front legs.
- The top of the head should be stripped short leaving hair on cheeks and under throat to form a ruff.
- Leave short padded brows.
- Undocked tails should be padded.

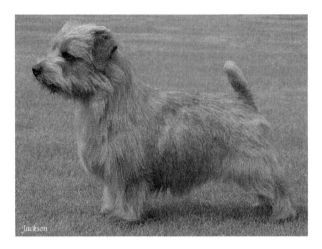

Fig. 11.69 Norfolk Terrier: Show dog. (Photo courtesy of John D. Jackson.)

Norwich Terrier (Te-Wi)

General appearance: Small, low, keen dog, compact and strong with good substance and bone. Honourable scars from wear and tear not to be unduly penalised.

Characteristics: One of the smallest of terriers. Loveable disposition, not quarrelsome, tremendously active with hardy constitution.

Recommended time between trims: 3–4 months.

Consult checklists in Chapter 10.

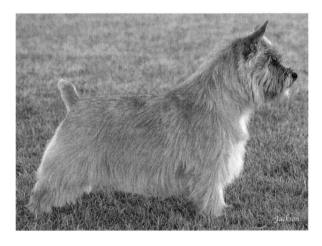

Fig. 11.70 Norwich Terrier: Show dog. (Photo courtesy of John D. Jackson.)

- The entire coat should be hand-stripped. However, if the skin is in poor condition or the coat is of poor texture hand-stripping may not always be appropriate as this could cause irritation.

- Using thinning scissors all over the coat will create a more natural look.
- Clipping the coat is not advisable as this would cut into the undercoat and leave marks.
- You can assess the readiness of the coat by how it stands away from the body and by gently pulling a few hairs. If the coat is tight to the body and the hair is difficult to pull out, it is not ready to strip.
- Leave a little feathering on the rear and front legs. The top of the head should be stripped short leaving hair on cheeks and under throat to form a ruff.
- Leave short padded brows.
- Undocked tails should be padded.

Old English Sheepdog (Pa-Dc2)

General appearance: Strong, square-looking dog with great symmetry and overall soundness. Absolutely free from legginess, profusely coated all over. A thickset, muscular, able-bodied dog with a most intelligent expression. The natural outline should not be artificially changed by scissoring or clipping.

Characteristics: Of great stamina, exhibiting a gently rising topline and a pear-shaped body when viewed from above. The gait has a typical roll when ambling or walking. Bark has a distinctive toned quality.

Recommended time between trims: 4–6 weeks.

Consult checklists in Chapter 10.

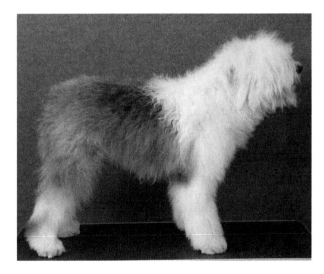

Fig. 11.71 Old English Sheepdog: Puppy.

- A full-coated Old English Sheepdog should only have the hygiene areas and under the pads clipped (Fig. 11.71).
- Most pet owners prefer the feet scissored round and a fringe cut into the top-knot. To trim the fringe, place your thumb onto the stop and comb a small

amount of coat forward and trim across from the outer corner of one eye to the outer corner of the other eye. Comb another section and trim the overhang.
- To take the coat down further you can layer the coat using thinning scissors. Lift one section of the coat at a time and layer, following the coat growth. Trim the edges of the legs to neaten and trim around the head shape.
- The coat may be scissored all over to any length (Fig. 11.72).
- To shorten further clip the body coat (following the West Highland White body lines) and scissor the legs.
- If badly matted the coat may require complete clipping.

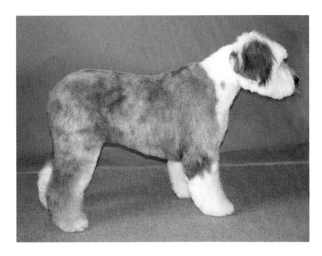

Fig. 11.72 Old English Sheepdog: Scissored down pet trim.

Papillion (To-Si)

General appearance: Dainty, well balanced little dog. An alert bearing and intelligent expression.
Characteristics: The name 'Papillion' is derived from the shape and position of the ears. When erect they are carried obliquely like the spread wings of a butterfly, hence the name. When the ears are completely dropped this type is known as the 'Phalene' (Moth). Head markings should be symmetrical, about a narrow white, clearly defined blaze which is desirable but not essential to represent the body of a butterfly.
Recommended time between trims: 3–4 months (but note: show dogs do not require trimming, only baths).
Consult checklists in Chapter 10.

- For show purposes no trimming is required.
- Most pet owners prefer feet trimmed to a natural style and hocks tidied.
- Thinning out of featherings around the rear and throat can be done with thinning scissors or a Coat King.

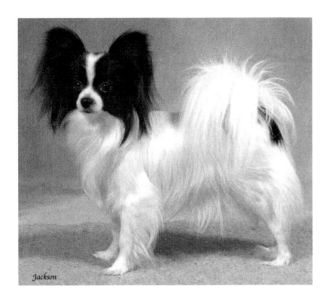

Fig. 11.73 Papillion: Show dog. (Photo courtesy of John D. Jackson.)

Parson Russell Terrier (Te-Wi)

General appearance: Workmanlike, active and agile; built for speed and endurance. Overall picture of balance and flexibility. Honourable scars permissible.

Characteristics: Essentially a working terrier with ability and conformation to go to ground and run with hounds.

Recommended time between trims: 3–4 months.

Consult checklists in Chapter 10.

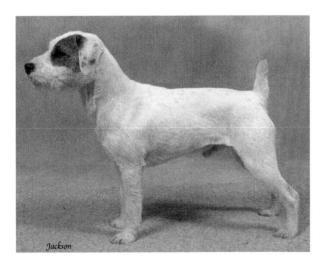

Fig. 11.74 Parson Russell Terrier: Show dog. (Photo courtesy of John D. Jackson.)

- The entire coat should be hand-stripped. However, if the skin is in poor condition or the coat is of poor texture hand-stripping may not always be appropriate as this could cause irritation.
- Using thinning scissors all over the coat will create a more natural look.
- Clipping the coat is not advisable as this would cut into the undercoat and leave marks.
- Leave slight padded brows and beard.

Pekingese (To-Dc1)

General appearance: Small, well balanced, thick set dog of dignity and quality.
Characteristics: Leonine in appearance with alert and intelligent expression.
Recommended time between trims: 3–4 months.
Consult checklists in Chapter 10.

- The show dog should not be trimmed.
- Many pet owners prefer feet trimmed in a natural style (Fig. 11.75).

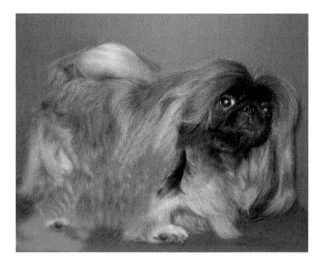

Fig. 11.75 Pekingese: Pet tidy in a natural style.

Polish Lowland Sheepdog (Pa-Dc2)

General appearance: Medium size, cobby, strong, muscular, fairly long, thick coat.
Characteristics: Lively but self-controlled, watchful, bright, clever, perceptive with excellent memory. Easy to train, works as a herding and watchdog.
Recommended time between trims: 4–8 weeks.
Consult checklists in Chapter 10.

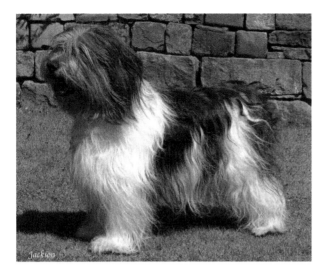

Fig. 11.76 Polish Lowland Sheepdog: Show dog. (Photo courtesy of John D. Jackson.)

- A full-coated Polish Lowland Sheepdog should only have the hygiene areas and under the pads clipped (Fig. 11.76).
- Most pet owners prefer the feet scissored round and a fringe cut into the top-knot. To trim the fringe, place your thumb onto the stop and comb a small amount of coat forward and trim across from the outer corner of one eye to the outer corner of the other eye. Comb another section and trim the overhang.
- To take the coat down further you can layer the coat using thinning scissors. Lift one section of the coat at a time and layer, following the coat growth. Trim the edges of the legs to neaten and trim around the head shape.
- The coat could be scissored all over to any required length.
- To shorten further clip the body coat (following the West Highland White body lines) and scissor the legs.
- If badly matted the coat may require complete clipping.

Pomeranian (To-Dc1)

General appearance: Compact, short-coupled dog, well knit in frame. Exhibiting great intelligence in expression; activity and buoyancy in deportment.
Characteristics: Sound, vivacious and dainty.
Recommended time between trims: 8–12 weeks.
Consult checklists in Chapter 10.

- Trim natural feet.
- Trim padded hocks.
- Scissor the ear tips.
- To create a circular-shaped dog place tail over back and trim all outer edges (Fig. 11.77).

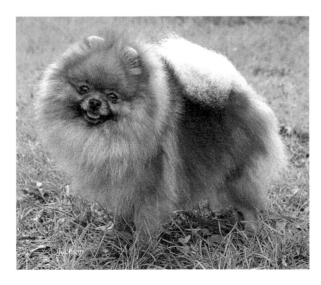

Fig. 11.77 Pomeranian: Show dog. (Photo courtesy of John D. Jackson.)

Poodle (Ut-Wo)

General appearance: Well balanced, elegant looking with very proud carriage.
Characteristics: Distinguished by a special type of clip for show activity and by a type of coat that does not moult.
Recommended time between trims: 4–6 weeks.
Consult checklists in Chapter 10.

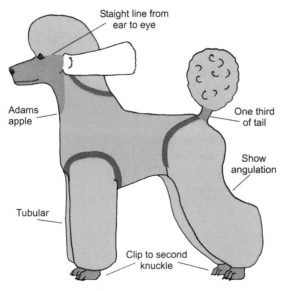

Scissors
Fine blade = 15 against the growth.
Medium blade = 5F
Blend with scissors
Untrimmed

Fig. 11.78 Poodle trim.

- The lion trim should be followed for show dogs.
- Most pet owners prefer a more practical style – the commonest being the lamb trim (Fig. 11.79).
- Variations can be a scissored face (Fig. 11.80), scissored body and scissored feet.
- Moustaches and beards can be left on a clipped face. To align correctly follow a diagonal line from the just above the nose to the canine tooth.

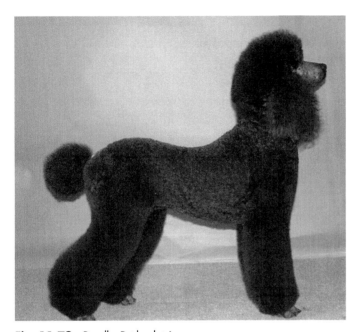

Fig. 11.79   Poodle: Pet lamb trim.

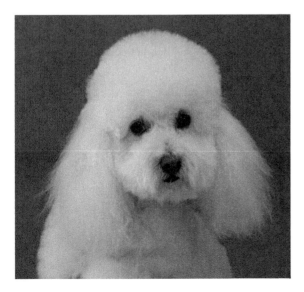

Fig. 11.80   Poodle: Pet scissored face.

Rough Collie (Pa-Dc1)

General appearance: Appears as dog of great beauty, standing with impassive dignity, with no part out of proportion to whole.

Characteristics: Physical structure on lines of strength and activity, free from cloddiness and no trace of coarseness. Expression most important. In considering relative values it is obtained by perfect balance and combination of skull and foreface, size, shape, colour and placement of eyes, correct position and carriage of ears.

Recommended time between trims: 3–4 months.

Consult checklists in Chapter 10.

- Trim natural feet.
- Trim padded hocks.
- Tidy area between main and stopper pad.

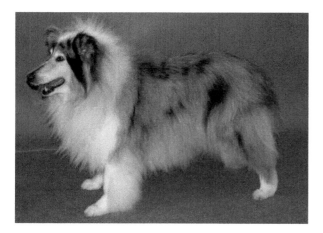

Fig. 11.81 Rough Collie: Pet tidy in a natural style.

Samoyed (Pa-Dc1)

General appearance: Most striking. Medium and well balanced. Strong, active and graceful, free from coarseness but capable of great endurance.

Characteristics: Intelligent, alert, full of action. 'Smiling expression'.

Recommended time between trims: 3–4 months.

Consult checklists in Chapter 10.

- Trim natural feet.
- Trim padded hocks.

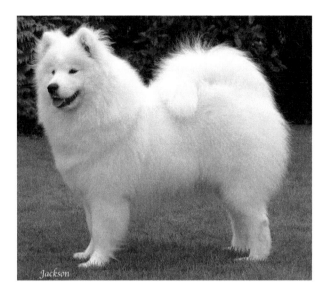

Fig. 11.82 Samoyed: Show dog. (Photo courtesy of John D. Jackson.)

Schnauzer (Ut-Wi)

General appearance: Sturdily built, robust, sinewy, nearly square (length of body equal to height at shoulders). Expression keen and attitude alert. Correct conformation is of more importance than colour or purely 'beauty' points.

Characteristics: Strong, vigorous dog capable of great endurance.

Recommended time between trims: 8–12 weeks.

Consult checklists in Chapter 10.

- The coat should be hand-stripped.
- The head, throat, chest and rear muscle should still be clipped.
- An undocked tail should be clipped short.

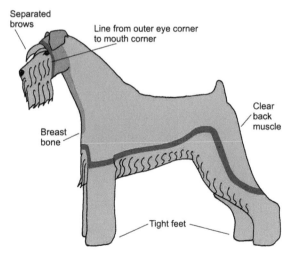

Scissors or thinning scissors
Fine blade = 10 with the growth or 7F against the growth. Ears 15.
Medium blade = 7F
Blend with thinning scissors

Separated brows

Line from outer eye corner to mouth corner

Clear back muscle

Breast bone

Tight feet

Fig. 11.83 Schnauzer.

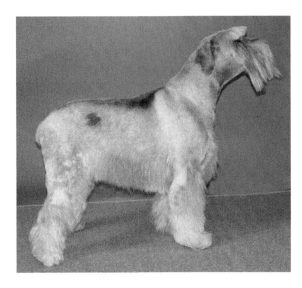

Fig. 11.84 Schnauzer: Clipped back pet trim.

Scottish Terrier (Te-Wi)

General appearance: Thick-set, of suitable size to go to ground, short-legged, alert in carriage and suggestive of great power and activity in small compass. Head gives impression of being long for size of dog. Very agile and active in spite of short legs.

Characteristics: Loyal and faithful. Dignified, independent and reserved, but courageous and highly intelligent.

Recommended time between trims: 8–12 weeks.

Consult checklists in Chapter 10.

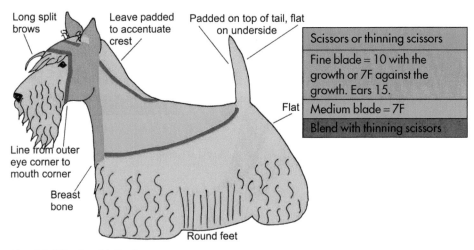

Fig. 11.85 Scottish Terrier.

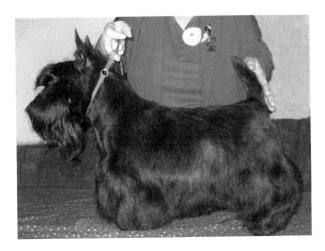

Fig. 11.86 Scottish Terrier: Hand-stripped pet trim.

- The body coat should be hand-stripped.
- You can assess the readiness of the coat by how it stands away from the body and by gently pulling a few hairs. If the coat is tight to the body and the hair is difficult to pull out, it is not ready to strip.
- The head, throat and chest should be clipped.
- Leave a tuft of hair on inside of corner of ear.

Sealyham Terrier (Te-Wi)

General appearance: Free moving, active, balanced and of great substance in small compass. General outline oblong, not square.
Characteristics: Sturdy, game and workmanlike.
Recommended time between trims: 8–12 weeks.
Consult checklists in Chapter 10.

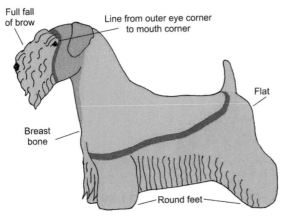

Scissors or thinning scissors
Fine blade = 10 with the growth or 7F against the growth. Ears 15.
Medium blade = 7F
Blend with thinning scissors

Fig. 11.87 Sealyham Terrier.

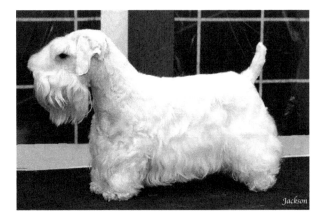

Fig. 11.88 Sealyham Terrier: Show dog. (Photo courtesy of John D. Jackson.)

- The body coat should be hand-stripped.
- You can assess the readiness of the coat by how it stands away from the body and by gently pulling a few hairs. If the coat is tight to the body and the hair is difficult to pull out, it is not ready to strip.
- The head and chest should be clipped.

Shetland Sheepdog (Pa-Dc1)

General appearance: Small, long-haired working dog of great beauty, free from cloddiness and coarseness. Outline symmetrical so that no part appears out of proportion to whole. Abundant coat, mane and frill, shapeliness of head and sweetness of expression combined to present the ideal.
Characteristics: Alert, gentle, intelligent, strong and active.
Recommended time between trims: 3–4 months.
Consult checklists in Chapter 10.

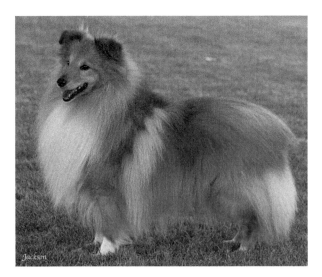

Fig. 11.89 Shetland Sheepdog: Show dog. (Photo courtesy of John D. Jackson.)

- Trim natural feet.
- Trim padded hocks.
- Tidy area between main and stopper pads.

Shih Tzu (Ut-Dc2)

General appearance: Sturdy, abundantly coated dog with distinctly arrogant carriage and chrysanthemum-like face.
Characteristics: Intelligent, active and alert.
Recommended time between trims: 4–8 weeks.
Consult checklists in Chapter 10.

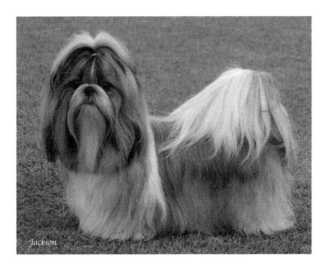

Fig. 11.90 Shih Tzu: Show dog. (Photo courtesy of John D. Jackson.)

- A full-coated Shih Tzu should only have the hygiene areas and under the pads clipped.
- For show purposes the top knot should be fastened (Fig. 11.90).
- Most pet owners prefer the feet scissored round and a fringe cut into the top-knot. To trim the fringe, place your thumb onto the stop and comb a small amount of coat forward and trim across from the outer corner of one eye to the outer corner of the other eye. Comb another section and trim the overhang.
- To take the coat down further you can layer the coat using thinning scissors. Lift one section of the coat at a time and layer, following the coat growth. Trim the edges of the legs to neaten and trim around the head shape.
- The coat could be scissored all over to any required length.
- To shorten further clip the body coat (following the West Highland White body lines) and scissor the legs.
- If badly matted the coat may require complete clipping.

Soft Coated Wheaten Terrier (Te-Si)

General appearance: Medium-sized, compact, understanding terrier well covered with a soft, wheaten-coloured, natural coat that falls in loose curves or waves. An active, short-coupled dog, strong and well built; well balanced in structure and movement, not exaggerated in any way. Standing fore square with head and tail up, giving the appearance of a happy dog, full of character.

Characteristics: A natural terrier with strong sporting instincts, hardy and of strong constitution.

Recommended time between trims: 4–6 weeks.

Consult checklists in Chapter 10.

- Tidy body and legs to accentuate shape.

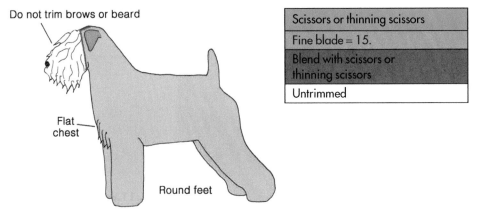

Scissors or thinning scissors
Fine blade = 15.
Blend with scissors or thinning scissors
Untrimmed

Fig. 11.91 Soft Coated Wheaten Terrier.

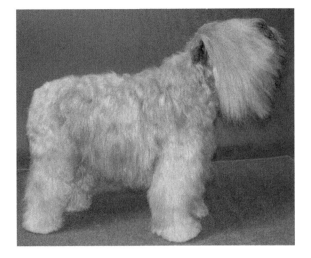

Fig. 11.92 Soft Coated Wheaten Terrier: Pet trim.

St. Bernard (Wo-Dc1)

General appearance: Well proportioned and of great substance.
Characteristics: Distinctly marked, large-sized, mountain-rescue dog.
Recommended time between trims: 3–4 months.
Consult checklists in Chapter 10.

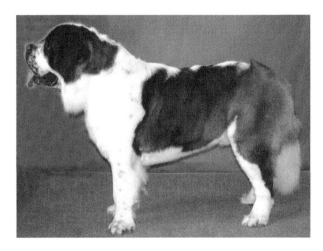

Fig. 11.93 St. Bernard: Pet tidy.

- For rough-coated, feet may be trimmed to natural style.
- Tidy the hocks.
- For pet purposes thinning of rear feathers can be done using thinners or a Coat King.

Sussex Spaniel (Gd-Si)

General appearance: Massive, strongly built. Active, energetic dog, whose characteristic movement is a decided roll, and unlike that of any other spaniel.
Characteristics: Natural working ability, gives tongue at work in thick cover.
Recommended time between trims: 8–12 weeks.
Consult checklists in Chapter 10.

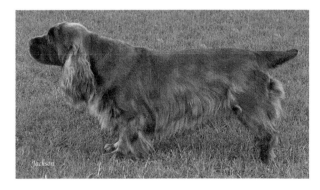

Fig. 11.94 Sussex Spaniel: Show dog. (Photo courtesy of John D. Jackson.)

- This coat should be hand-stripped unless the dog has been neutered (see below). Remove dull, fluffy coat with finger and thumb. If the coat lies flat naturally do not clip unless requested by the owner.
- A neutered dog may have a very fluffy, pale coloured coat. Clipping is often the only option for these dogs and hand-stripping would not be successful.
- Trim natural feet.
- Trim padded hocks.
- An undocked tail should be trimmed in a flag shape.
- The overall effect should be natural and flowing.

Tibetan Terrier (Ut-Dc2)

General appearance: Sturdy, medium-sized, long-haired, generally square outline. Balanced, without exaggeration.
Characteristics: Lively, good-natured. Loyal companion dog with many engaging ways.
Recommended time between trims: 4–6 weeks.
Consult checklists in Chapter 10.

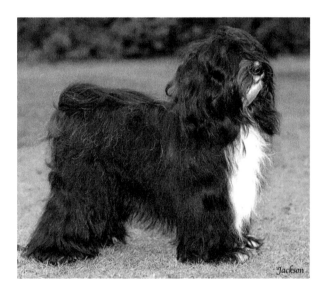

Fig. 11.95 Tibetan Terrier: Show dog. (Photo courtesy of John D. Jackson.)

- A full-coated Tibetan Terrier should only have the hygiene areas and under the pads clipped (Fig. 11.95).
- Most pet owners prefer the feet scissored round and a fringe cut into the topknot. To trim the fringe, place your thumb onto the stop and comb a small amount of coat forward and trim across from the outer corner of one eye to the outer corner of the other eye. Comb another section and trim the overhang.

- To take the coat down further you can layer the coat using thinning scissors. Lift one section of the coat at a time and layer, following the coat growth. Trim the edges of the legs to neaten and trim around the head shape.
- The coat could be scissored all over to any required length.
- To shorten further clip the body coat (following the West Highland White body lines) and scissor the legs (Fig. 11.96).
- If badly matted the coat may require complete clipping.
- Finish the head in a 'teddy-bear' trim.

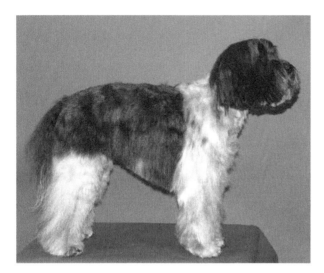

Fig. 11.96 Tibetan Terrier: Shortened pet trim.

Welsh Springer Spaniel (Gd-Si)

General appearance: Symmetrical, compact, not leggy, obviously built for endurance and hard work. Quick and active mover, displaying plenty of push and drive.

Characteristics: Very ancient and distinct breed of pure origin. Strong, merry and very active.

Recommended time between trims: 8–12 weeks.

Consult checklists in Chapter 10.

- The body coat should lay flat. Use finger and thumb, stripping knife or Coat King to remove straggly ends.
- DO NOT clip body coat. This will ruin colour and texture.
- Trim natural feet.
- Trim padded hocks.
- Tidy area between main and stopper pad.
- Feathering should be natural and flowing.
- Strip, thin or clip excessive coat on the ears depending on density.
- Thin out excessive coat on throat.

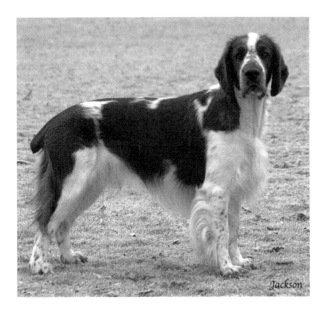

Fig. 11.97 Welsh Springer Spaniel: Show dog. (Photo courtesy of John D. Jackson.)

Welsh Terrier (Te-Wi)

General appearance: Smart, workmanlike, well balanced and compact.
Characteristics: Affectionate, obedient and easily controlled.
Recommended time between trims: 8–12 weeks.
Consult checklists in Chapter 10.

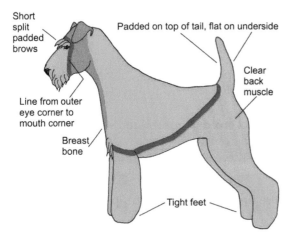

Short split padded brows

Padded on top of tail, flat on underside

Clear back muscle

Line from outer eye corner to mouth corner

Breast bone

Tight feet

Scissors or thinning scissors
Fine blade = 10 with the growth or 7F against the growth. Ears 15.
Medium blade = 7F
Blend with thinning scissors

Fig. 11.98 Welsh Terrier.

- This breed is normally hand-stripped for the show ring.
- You can assess the readiness of the coat by how it stands away from the body and by gently pulling a few hairs. If the coat is tight to the body and the hair is difficult to pull out, it is not ready to strip.

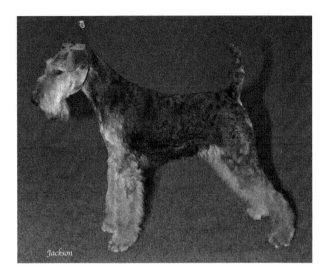

Fig. 11.99 Welsh Terrier: Show dog. (Photo courtesy of John D. Jackson.)

West Highland White Terrier (Te-Wi)

General appearance: Strongly built; deep in chest and back ribs; level back and powerful quarters on muscular legs and exhibiting to a marked degree a great combination of strength and activity.

Characteristics: Small, active, game, hardy, possessed of no small amount of self-esteem with a varminty appearance.

Recommended time between trims: 8–12 weeks.

Consult checklists in Chapter 10.

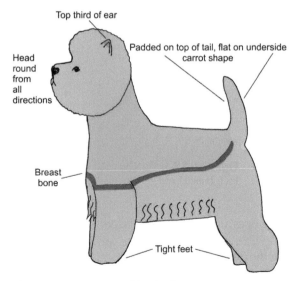

Scissors or thinning scissors		
Fine blade = 10		
Medium blade = 5F		
Blend with thinning scissors		

Top third of ear

Head round from all directions

Padded on top of tail, flat on underside carrot shape

Breast bone

Tight feet

Fig. 11.100 West Highland White Terrier.

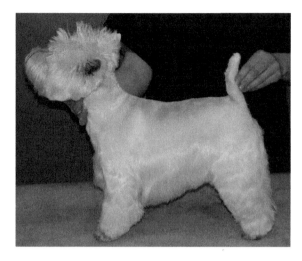

Fig. 11.101 West Highland White Terrier: Clipped back pet trim.

- This breed is normally hand-stripped for the show ring.
- You can assess the readiness of the coat by how it stands away from the body and by gently pulling a few hairs. If the coat is tight to the body and the hair is difficult to pull out, it is not ready to strip.
- For pet purposes the coat can be clipped (Fig. 11.101).

Pet head trim

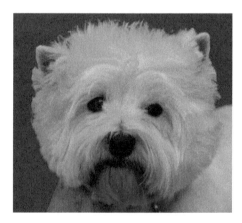

Fig. 11.102 West Highland White Terrier: Pet trimmed head.

- Trim the hair in the corners of the eyes with thinning scissors – do not over trim here.
- Trim a fringe to create a visor over the eyes.
- The head should be a circular shape and all the hair the same length.

- Scissor a semi-circle outline from the nose to behind the ear – the longest point being below the eye.
- Comb hair back and tidy any overhang at the back of the neck and ears with thinning scissors.
- Lift the hair on top of the head and sides in sections using thinning scissors to create a circular shape (a layered full appearance).

Wire Fox Terrier (Te-Wi)

General appearance: Active and lively, bone and strength in small compass, never cloddy or coarse. Conformation to show perfect balance; in particular this applies to the relative proportions of skull and foreface, and similarly height at withers and length of body from shoulder point to buttocks appear approximately equal. Standing like a short-backed hunter, covering a lot of ground.
Characteristics: Alert, quick of movement, keen of expression, on tiptoe of expectation at the slightest provocation.
Recommended time between trims: 8–12 weeks.
Consult checklists in Chapter 10.

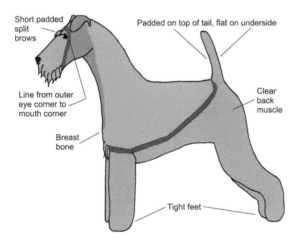
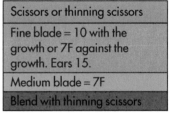

Fig. 11.103 Wire Fox Terrier.

- This breed is normally hand-stripped for the show ring.
- You can assess the readiness of the coat by how it stands away from the body and by gently pulling a few hairs. If the coat is tight to the body and the hair is difficult to pull out, it is not ready to strip.

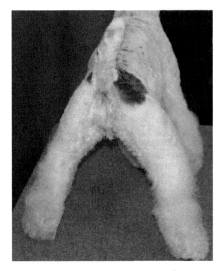

Fig. 11.104 Wire Fox Terrier: Shows rear trimming.

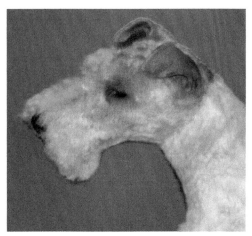

Fig. 11.105 Wire Fox Terrier: Pet trimmed head.

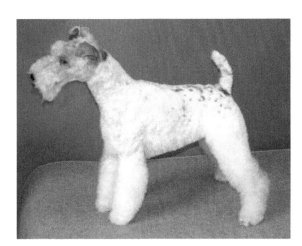

Fig. 11.106 Wire Fox Terrier: Clipped pet body.

Yorkshire Terrier (To-Si)

General appearance: Long coated, coat hanging quite straight and evenly down each side, parting extending from nose to end of tail. Very compact and neat, carriage very upright conveying an important air. General outline conveying impression of vigorous and well-proportioned body.

Characteristics: Alert, intelligent toy terrier.

Recommended time between trims: 6–12 weeks.

Consult checklists in Chapter 10.

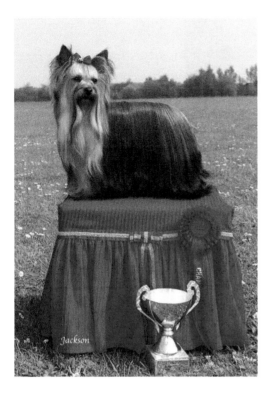

Fig. 11.107 Yorkshire Terrier: Show dog. (Photo courtesy of John D. Jackson.)

- For show purposes the top knot should be fastened with the coat long and flowing (Fig. 11.107).
- A full-coated Yorkshire Terrier should only have the hygiene areas under the pads and tips of the ears clipped.
- Most pet owners prefer the feet scissored round and a fringe cut into the topknot. To trim the fringe, place your thumb onto the stop and comb a small amount of coat forward and trim across from the outer corner of one eye to the outer corner of the other eye. Comb another section and trim the overhang.
- To take the coat down further you can layer the coat using thinning scissors. Lift one section of the coat at a time and layer, following the coat growth. Trim the edges of the legs to neaten and trim around the head shape.
- To shorten further clip the body coat (following the West Highland White body lines) and scissor the legs (Figs 11.108 and 11.109).
- Some fine-textured coats are suitable to use thinning scissors to shorten the back coat.
- If badly matted the coat may require complete clipping.

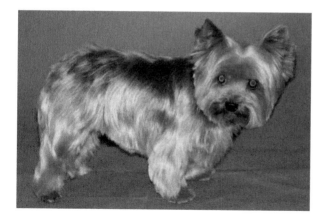

Fig. 11.108 Yorkshire Terrier: Clipped body pet trim.

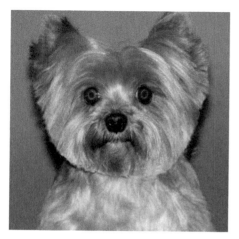

Fig. 11.109 Yorkshire Terrier: West Highland style head.

CROSSBREEDS

These can have any of the coat types or a combination of coat types and colours. Many dogs that visit a grooming salon are crossbreeds, varying from first cross (both parents are known) to multi-cross (parentage unknown).

Many crossbreeds may have specific names, e.g. Patterdale Terrier, Fell Terrier and Labradoodle to mention a few. Remember that these dogs may vary in coat type so do not assume that two Patterdales or Labradoodles are the same.

When deciding how best to trim a crossbreed, take into account:

- Its characteristics
- Its coat type
- The owner's wishes

Use your knowledge of styling specific breeds and adapt styles for the cross-breed. Do not be afraid to mix and match styles, e.g. a West Highland White (Te-Wi) trim may suit a dog's body and legs but if it has dropped ears an Airedale (Te-Wi) head may suit its head better.

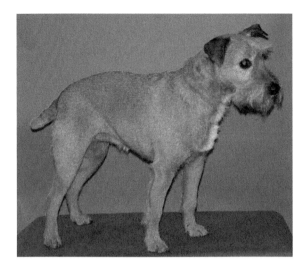

Fig. 11.110 Cross Breed: Hand-stripped Border Terrier style.

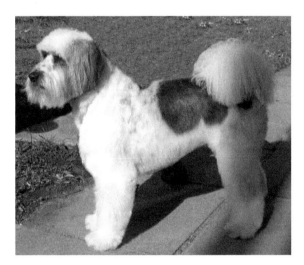

Fig. 11.111 Cross Breed: Teddy bear style.

Associations and events

Associations

British Dog Groomers Association
petcare.org.uk

English Groomers Group
englishgroomersgroup.org

Irish Professional Dog Groomers Association
ipdga.com

British Isles Grooming Association
britishislesgroomingassociation.org

Qualifications

The qualifications recognised by the Grooming Industry are the City and Guilds Level 2 Grooming Assistant, Level 3 Introductory Certificate, Level 3 Professional Diploma and LCGI.
cityandguilds.com

Other qualifications such as ICMG are also available.
icmguk.com

Higher Diploma Exam
petcare.org.uk

Dog Shows

For keeping ahead of the latest trends in breed styling there are many dog shows around the Country which can be a good source of information. The major event is Crufts which is held in March each year.
crufts.org.uk

For information on other shows go to fossedata.co.uk

Grooming Competitions

Master Groom International Grooming Competition.
mastergroom.org

English Groomers Group Challenge.
englishgroomersgroup.org

Premier Groom Grooming Competition.
premiergroom.co.uk

Northern Groomers
no direct web site available

British Grooming Championships
petcare.org

Educational Events are run throughout the year by various groups. Groom Team England has a dairy page on the web site *groomteamengland.com* with dates of some of these events, however the best place to find out about forthcoming events is face book.

Education and Training

City & Guilds directly or any City & Guilds approved centres.

Websites of interest to groomers

The National Register of Groomers, *igroomdogs.co.uk,* is a not-for-profit community which is hosted by the Animal Care College. This site helps to provide the best guidance for the owners of the UK's pets that require professional grooming.

Groomers Gallery

Grooming and breed trimming information is in association with the English Groomers Group.
groomersgallery.com

INDEX

Printed and bound by CPI Group (UK) Ltd, Croydon, CR0 4YY

27/10/2024

14580388-0002